Being Human
Ordinariness in Nursing

610·730699 TAY

WITHDRAWN

Being Human
Ordinariness in Nursing

Beverley J. Taylor RN RM PhD
Professor of Nursing, Southern Cross University, New South Wales

LIBRARY
LOTHIAN COLLEGE OF HEALTH STUDIES
23 CHALMERS STREET
EDINBURGH
EH3 9EW

LIBRARY	LOTHIAN COLLEGE OF HEALTH STUDIES
CLASS	W Y 87
ACC No.	14230
DATE	5/9/94
PRICE	10·45 ·

CHURCHILL LIVINGSTONE
MELBOURNE EDINBURGH LONDON MADRID NEW YORK AND TOKYO 1994

CHURCHILL LIVINGSTONE
Medical Division of Longman Group UK Limited

Distributed in Australia by Longman Cheshire Pty Limited,
Longman House, Kings Gardens, 95 Coventry Street, South
Melbourne 3205, and by associated companies, branches and
representatives throughout the world with the exception of Canada
and the United States of America.

© Beverley J. Taylor

All rights reserved. No part of this publication may be reproduced,
stored in a retrieval system, or transmitted in any form or by any
means, electronic, mechanical, photocopying, recording or
otherwise, without the prior permission of the publishers
(Churchill Livingstone, Robert Stevenson House, 1-3 Baxter's
Place, Leith Walk, Edinburgh EH1 3AF), or a licence permitting
restricted copying in the United Kingdom issued by the Copyright
Licensing Agency Ltd, 90 Tottenham Court Road, London, W1P
9HE.

First published 1994

ISBN   0-443-04952-1

National Library of Australia Cataloguing in Publication Data

Taylor, Beverley.
  Being human: ordinariness in nursing

  Bibliography.
  Includes index.
  ISBN 0 443 04952 1.

  1. Nursing - Practice. 2. Nurshing - Philosophy. 3. Nurse and
patient. 4. Communication in nursing. I. Title.

610.730699

Produced by Churchill Livingstone in Australia
Printed in Malaysia—VVP

For Churchill Livingstone in Melbourne
Publisher: Judy Waters
Co-ordinating Editor: Maja Ingrassia
Copy Editor: John Macdonald
Desktop Preparation: Sandra Tolra
Typesetting: Designpoint
Indexer: Master Indexing
Production Control: Peter Hylands
Design: Churchill Livingstone

The
publisher's
policy is to use
paper manufactured
from sustainable forests

Contents

Considerations

1. Nursing as a human relationship

Essentially, being human is about living in the world of other people and things. Although existence alone is not impossible if one could imagine oneself as living as a single identity in sublime isolation, reliant on no person or no thing, it must be accepted that, even in the most fundamental sense, human existence is related to finding oneself in the meshwork of one's own life, and its relationship to other people and things. Human life is complex potentially, because it involves a multiplicity of relationships that involve interactions with other people and things. We cannot help but take account of one another as we move around in our daily spheres of activity, extending our awareness beyond that which involves our inner and outer senses of our own bodies. We are social entities inevitably, given our interrelatedness to other people and things around us.

Nursing is a people-oriented vocation, involving all of the usual complexities of interhuman relationships, intensified even more by the extra effects of illness and the need for nursing care. Nurses are in unique positions, as people who have special knowledge and skills about other people and their responses to illness, and because they have front row seats to watch the dance of humanity; and, as such, they have the potential to make sense of human existence through close interactions with humans in need of care. If nurses begin to appreciate their potential for understanding interpersonal relationships, they may come to understand themselves as humans who share commonalities with the people in their care. In this way, nurses may begin to understand nursing itself, so that long-sought-after quest of nurses to define nursing as a human endeavour may be accomplished at last.

Nursing happens whenever nurses and patients are together in contexts of care; it is about how nurses and patients relate to one another to work through the circumstances that have brought them together as nurses and patients. As a human relationship, nursing

3

is made therapeutic by the humanness of interpersonal encounters. Those nurses who are able to acknowledge and value their own humanness in their professional lives bring a special gift to people in caring contexts, because they bring themselves as knowledgeable and skilful humans who are able to transcend the professional inhibitions of their roles to be 'just themselves.' Patients recognise and respect nurses' knowledge and skills and they trust in these professional prerequisites, but they are pleased when they find that nurses are humans, just like themselves. It is this affinity as humans, this thing that I have called 'ordinariness,' that allows nurses and patients to acknowledge each other as humans and to share in the transitory imposition of illness. Ordinariness in nursing makes the nurse-patient relationship therapeutic, so that healing occurs, and patients feel that their time spent in the health care facility has been made manageable by its familiarity as a human place.

This book will provide an explanation of the methods and insights that lead me to describe the phenomenon of ordinariness in nursing, as I witnessed it in a Professorial Nursing Unit in Australia. This book intends to be a reader-friendly version of my PhD thesis, and as such, it tells the story of how I became interested in the area of study, and how I went about finding a way of bringing out the nature and effects of the phenomenon, so that nursing itself, would benefit from the insights. I regard nursing as being that which happens between nurses and patients in contexts of care, and on this basic assumption I make my claim that the insights of this research have the potential of benefiting nurses and patients, by enriching their relationships in nursing practice settings.

Nursing is searching for ways of describing itself, and the way in which I have described nursing may seem simplistic to some people. Nursing has failed to express itself through complex descriptions, and it seems to me that just as the most sophisticated things are open to simple explanations, so are the nature and purposes of nursing. From some of the nursing literature it becomes evident that nurses have attempted to define nursing in terms of its tasks and role responsibilities, and all of these definitions have resulted in a sense of frustration from incompleteness, because none of them has managed successfully to convey the breadth and depth of nursing's span.

Nursing has attempted to define itself through expressing its human concerns, and these have been conveyed by epistemological and ontological means. Essentially, epistemology and ontology respectively refer to knowing and being as ways of understanding our world and our relationships to ourselves and other people and things in our world. At this point, it seems advantageous to give a simple description of being and knowing as human concerns, before reviewing some of the ways in which nursing scholars have represented nursing's existence and knowledge forms. The chapter will then describe nursing as that which happens between nurses and patients in contexts of care and, lastly, it will introduce the research relating to ordinariness in nursing.

Being and knowing as human concerns

Humans are curious about their own nature and existence and how this in turn relates to the existence of other people and things around them. Seeking to find answers for the questions related to how people live in the world, and thereby make sense of their existence as beings, is the quest of ontology. Human beings have a time honoured tradition of trying to understand what constitutes truth and, therefore, what counts as knowledge about themselves and their world; such revelations are the quest of epistemology.

Questions of ontology (Being) may be considered as related to questions of epistemology (knowing). Human existence and interpersonal interaction can be understood ontologically and epistemologically, by paying attention to the ways in which people make sense of their own human nature and to the ways in which they form and question the knowledge bases of human and environmental phenomena. That Being and knowing are not necessarily separate human concerns is the contention of some philosophers, such as Heidegger (1962) and Gadamer (1975), who connected ontology and epistemology as interdependent concerns. For them, answers about the nature of Being (with a capital B to denote the ontological nature of existence) automatically inform seekers of truth about the nature of knowledge. In their shared view, ontological questions raise epistemological answers because ontological answers create clearer and clearer explanations of existence and, as the ground of all things, finer and finer inextricable associations with existence itself, lead to clearer and clearer explanations of knowledge.

Ontology seeks to explicate the nature of people and things. The term 'ontology' is derived from *logos* (an account) and *onta* (of the Being of beings). Ontology is defined as:

> the theory of existence or, more narrowly, of what really is, as opposed to that which appears to exist but does not, or to that which

can properly be said to exist but if only conceived as some complex whose constituents are the things that really exist (Bullock Stallybrass & Trombley 1988 p605)

Accounting for the Being of beings has been a task of philosophy since the earliest philosophers, such as Parmenides, mused about the nature of existence. Ontological questions are posed about the nature of existence in terms of differences between appearances and reality, and philosophers have approached ontology from various perspectives to find these answers (Palmer 1988).

Epistemology seeks to validate the legitimacy of truth claims, thus philosophers have tackled rigorously epistemological problems encompassing questions about the origins, presuppositions, nature, extent and veracity of knowledge. Knowledge has been variously defined (in Angeles 1981 p143). For Plato there were two general realms of knowledge: the non-natural realm of Eternal Ideal Forms (Ideas) that are transcendent, unchanging, perfect, intelligible with certainty; and the natural realm of ordinary sensations and particular things that are temporal, changing, unstable, unintelligible, and uncertain.

In contrast to Plato, Aristotle divided knowledge into three parts: theoretical or the first philosophy; practical or praxis; and productive or poiesis/poietikos. Aristotle (in Angeles 1981 p142) claimed that:

> Only knowledge in the form of things can be directly known by reason (the intellect)...Knowledge is based on a process of uninferred experience or perception (intuitive induction) that grasps the necessary connections among the forms in the particular things experienced. This process provides the self-evident axioms, or first principles, for demonstrative knowledge; the organised deductive system called science.

Knowledge acquisition has been characterised by peaks and troughs, in that it experienced acceleration between 650 and 250 BC in the time of the ancient Greek philosophers (who provided the seeds of scientific thought) and went into decline in the Middle Ages from 500 to 1200 AD (Singer 1959). During a resurgence of interest in epistemological enquiry after the Middle Ages, Descartes (1970 trans.) considered that the quest was for 'universal wisdom' and that for things to be considered as truth, they needed to be certain and evident, thereby beyond doubt and improbability.

Knowledge generation throughout history has undergone changes that have been grouped into ways of knowing. The deductive, absolute and objective notions of scientific knowledge as proposed by Aristotle and Descartes were reinforced by Locke and Hume, who emphasised the need for logic and empiricism in forming relationships among ideas. This type of knowledge is the a posteriori form, which is empirical, inductive, scientific, and verifiable and comes from sense experience, unlike the a priori knowledge of which Kant (1929 trans.) spoke, which comes prior to and independent of sense experience. A priori knowledge is connected with concepts such as being necessary, certain, definitional, deductive, universally true, innate, and intuitive.

In more recent times, Habermas (1972) coined the term 'knowledge-constitutive interests' to refer to three distinct paradigms, which reflected his belief that knowledge is the outcome of human needs and interests. In his view, technical interest creates instrumental knowledge of causal explanation, which is mediated through work and forms the empirical-analytic or natural sciences. Practical interest creates practical understanding through the medium of language and forms the hermeneutic or 'interpretive' sciences. Emancipatory interest creates liberatory knowledge by reflection through the medium of power and forms the critical social sciences. Beyond Habermas, epistemology stretches itself towards the 21st century, through the modernist and postmodernist eras, dissolving the borders of knowledge categories, and attesting to the boundless and indescribable nature and potential of human knowing.

Nursing understood through Being

Being and knowing are concerns of being human, and, by connections with the human relationships in nursing, they are a means of understanding the nature and effects of nursing.

If nursing is considered ontologically, the nature of nursing can be made manifest by locating and describing the nature of some nurse-patient relationships as they are lived out daily between nurses and patients. Using this perspective, the nature of Being is understood as the lived experience of nursing, which relates, in turn, to knowing the nature and effects of nursing.

In generating their accounts of the Being of beings in nursing, scholars have attempted to describe nursing by describing metaparadigm concepts of person, health, environment and nursing (Fawcett 1989). Of particular interest in conceptualising Being, as it is manifested in nursing, are scholars' descriptions of the person and nursing. Patients and nurses are beings, who embody Being; that is, they are entities within whom existence is situated. In this sense, 'Being-in-nursing' is 'what really is' in nursing; that is, it is the nurse-patient relationship as it is lived in health care contexts. The meaning of nursing is embodied in nurses and patients, and it is manifested by them, as they interact daily together.

Nursing occurs in social contexts, in which intersubjective meanings are generated. With encouragement from nursing scholars (Allen 1985, Allen, Benner & Diekelmann 1986, Benner 1984, 1985, Benner & Wrubel 1989, Carper 1978, Chinn 1988, Davis 1973, 1978, Field & Morse 1985, Parse 1987, Thompson 1987, Watson 1981) to express their experience of nursing in alternative ways, nurses have attempted to describe nursing from the intersubjective viewpoints of its participants.

A growing body of literature, using interpretive approaches to understanding the lived experiences of nurses and patients, attests to nurses' responsiveness in shifting from exclusive, postivistically-oriented understandings of nursing (Anderson 1981, 1987, Banonis 1989, Benner 1984, Benner & Wrubel 1989, Brown 1986, Drew 1986, Forrest 1989, Gulino 1982, Hyde 1977, Kretlow 1989–1990, McMahon & Pearson 1990, McPherson 1987, Mitchell 1990, Parse 1990, Paterson 1971, 1978, Paterson & Zderad 1976, Watson 1985).

In agreement with the definition of lived experience given by Dilthey (1985), Dreyfus (1979 in Benner & Wrubel 1989 p83) claimed that '[w]e are able to move around in the everyday world because our understanding is always situated and our actions are typically only as orderly as the situation demands.' Using some explanations given by Heidegger and Dreyfus, Benner and Wrubel (1989 p82) claimed that the lived experience of nursing involves a level of involvement and absorption in the situation, because 'there can be no situationless involvement'. For these scholars, the context of nursing requires an appreciation of the value of lived experience.

Contextually appropriate understandings and actions have been described by Benner and Wrubel (1989 p412), who extended the general meaning of 'environment' as it is defined in nursing literature, to refer to 'situation,' which implies 'the relevant concerns, issues, information, constraints, and resources at a given span of time or place as experienced by particular persons.' It becomes apparent by this redefinition, therefore, that the way nurses and patients make sense of their situations will be 'in terms of their own personal concerns, background meanings, temporality, habitual, cultural bodies, emotions and reflective thoughts' (p82). The lived experience of nursing, therefore, connects nurses and patients inextricably with the people and things in their worlds, not only as people engaged in present dialogue, but also as people who embody their past and anticipate their future.

Paterson and Zderad formulated a humanistic nursing model after a number of years in clinical practice and teaching, during which they identified the inability of positivistic science to address phenomena in nursing relating to nursing settings and the nature of people within them. Based on the phenomenological perspectives of Husserl, Marcel, and Buber, they developed the construct of nursology, using phenomenological methods to pose questions and search for answers about nursing. Paterson and Zderad (1976 p19) conceptualised nursing as:

a lived act, a response to a human situation. The response is purposely directed toward nurturing the well-being and more-being of a person with perceived needs related to the illness/health quality of living.

In seeking to explicate an existential, phenomenological view of nursing, Paterson and Zderad (1976 p51) described humanistic nursing as:

the act of nursing, the intersubjective transactional relation, the dialogue experience, lived in concert between persons where comfort and nurturance prod mutual unfolding.

In attesting to the value of the lived experience of people in their worlds, nursing scholars (Benner 1984, Benner & Wrubel 1989, Kestenbaum 1982, Munhall & Oiler 1986, Oiler 1982, 1986, Parse 1981, 1985, 1987, Paterson 1971, 1978, Paterson & Zderad 1976) have written about the lived experience of nursing. An humanistic nursing perspective is phenomenological essentially, in the sense that it attests to the meaning people find in their worlds; however, whereas some humanistic perspectives are unarguably interpretive in intent, if they do not seek to explicate the Being of beings in nursing, they cannot, with methodological accuracy, be termed phenomenological.

Benner (1984) was influenced by phenomenological perspectives of experience (Heidegger 1962 trans., Gadamer 1975 trans.), and by notions of expert practice (Dreyfus & Dreyfus 1980), to describe the knowledge embedded in expert nursing practice. Using paradigm cases around patient care issues, Benner (1984 p11) was able to define nursing practice at all levels of sophistication from novice to expert and conclude that:

a wealth of untapped knowledge is embedded in the practices and the 'know-how' of expert nurse clinicians, but this knowledge will not expand or fully develop unless nurses systematically record what they learn from their own experience.

Benner (1984) was speaking of the lived experience of practice as a way of knowing in nursing. Benner and Wrubel (1989 p7) took a phenomenological stance based on the work of Heidegger (1962 trans.) and Merleau-Ponty (1962) and focussed 'on the lived experiences of being healthy and being ill.' They claimed that:

[t]he best nursing practitioners understand the differences and relationships among health, illness and disease. This understanding leads nurses to seek the patient's story in formal and informal nursing histories, because they know that every illness has a story—plans that are threatened or thwarted, relationships are disturbed, and symptoms become laden with meaning depending on what else is happening in the person's life...(Benner & Wrubel 1989 p9)

In summary, the nursing literature attempts to understand the Being of beings (the existence of entities) in nursing, through descriptions of the metaparadigm concepts of person and nursing, and in written accounts of the lived experiences of nurses and patients in their respective contexts. Describing the lived experiences of nurses and patients is a rich area that promises to offer up deep insights into understanding nursing as it is lived in the ordinary day to day lives of nurses and patients.

Nursing understood through knowing

Knowing in nursing reflects the epistemological debates of philosophers. In this section, knowing in nursing will be addressed from the perspectives of some nurse scholars, who have attempted to define nursing (Abdellah et al 1960, Benner 1984, Benner & Wrubel 1989, Frederick & Northam 1938, Henderson 1955, King 1971, Kinlein 1977, Nightingale 1893, Orem 1959, Orlando 1961, Paterson & Zderad 1976, Peplau 1952, Rogers 1961, Roy 1976, Travelbee 1971, Wiedenbach 1964) and by the work of others, who have described nursing in terms of possible epistemological categories (Allen Benner & Diekelmann 1986, Carper 1978, Chinn & Kramer 1991, Parse 1987).

Epistemological considerations in nursing can be traced through the writings of scholars in nursing. One of the aims of epistemology in nursing has been to define nursing itself. Nurses have not reached a consensus on an accepted definition of nursing, reflecting possibly the diverse understandings of nurses of their experiences, and the tendency of classic definitions of nursing to reveal some epistemological aspects of nursing through the lenses of their unique sociocultural histories.

Notwithstanding a lack of definitional consensus, Erickson, Tomlin and Swain (1983 p29) found commonalities in what nurses say collectively, with themes being evident of the mission of nursing to:

assist persons; with their responses to health and illness states; with their self-care practices in relation to their health (with their coping and adapting); to achieve a state of (optimum) wellness by way of an interpersonal process.

A classic definition of nursing was given by Nightingale (1893 in Seymer 1955 pp334-335), who believed that:

[nursing puts] us in the best possible conditions for Nature to restore or to preserve health—to prevent or to cure disease or injury. Health is not only to be well but to be able to use well every power we have to use...Partly, perhaps mainly, upon nursing must depend whether Nature succeeds or fails in her attempt to cure by sickness. Nursing is therefore to help the patient to live...Nursing is an art, and an art requiring an organised practical and scientific training.

Nightingale recognised that living in her era, and her immediate future, meant that nursing required scientific legitimacy and she cleverly placed nursing in the scientific arena and connected the art and science of nursing. For Nightingale, the doing of nursing required practical and technical knowledge, the latter guiding the art of practice.

In extending the notion of supporting Nature, and in keeping with the emphasis on technical knowledge generated at that time by the empirico-analytical methods of science, Frederick and Northam (1938 p3) claimed that:

[n]ursing requires the application of scientific knowledge and nursing skills and affords the opportunities for constructive work in the care and relief of patients and their families...Modern nursing is by no means limited to giving of expert physical care to the sick, important as this is. It is more far reaching, including as it does, helping the patient adjust to unalterable situations, such as personal, family and economic conditions, teaching him and others in the home and in the community to care for themselves, guiding him in the prevention of illness through hygienic living, and helping him to use the available community resources to these ends.

Nursing here was described in terms of its role of helping individuals to help themselves, thus knowing nursing, at this point in time, involved seeing health as not facilitated solely by Nature and the nurse, but also by the community supports and the indi
tendency to seek them.

Peplau (1952 p16) described nursing as 'a significant, thera-peutic, interpersonal process.' The nurse was viewed as a member of the health care team. Unlike Nightingale, and Frederick and Northam, Peplau did not assume that nurses were the only people capable of knowing how to care for the sick. For Peplau, the role of nursing was shared by other health professionals, and their approaches to caring as an underpinning knowledge base had an influence on nursing, as evidenced by the outcome oriented language: 'Nursing is an educative instrument'. There was a mixture of caring and controlling, a struggle of sorts between the scientific and interpretive ways of knowing in vogue in nursing at that time.

Henderson agreed with her contemporaries that knowing in nursing was about helping people to help themselves, and this theme persisted in nursing definitions. A classic definition of nursing attributed to Henderson (1955 p4) was that:

[n]ursing is primarily assisting the individual (sick or well) in the performance of those activities contributing to health, or its recovery (or to a peaceful death) that he would perform unaided if he had the necessary strength, will, or knowledge.

Orem (1959) and Kinlein (1977) built on the concept of self-care, putting the responsibility back into the hands of the person receiving care, with the nurse giving assistance only as it was required. It is interesting to note that, as early as the late 1950's, nursing was known as facilitative of patient self-care activities, even though those self-care practices are still being realised partially in actual clinical areas. Nurses tend to want to do things for people, rather than to allow them to take time to do it for themselves. The apparent lack of congruency between clinical ideals and realities is highlighted by this way of knowing nursing.

Abdellah, Beland, Martin and Matheney (1960 p24) connected the notions of the knowledge base and the service of nursing and claimed that:

[n]ursing is a service to individuals and to families; therefore, to society. It is based upon an art and science which mold the attitudes, intellectual competencies, and technical skills of the individual nurse into the desire and ability to help people, sick or well, cope with their health needs, and may be carried out under general or specific medical direction.

It is interesting to note the inclusion in this definition of the accountability of nurses to doctors. The role of the doctor in the health care hierarchy was acknowledged, although not addressed, as were the potential tensions between nurses and doctors in relation to how they might know their respective worlds as products of their personal and professional sociocultural histories.

Orlando (1961), Rogers (1961) and Wiedenbach (1964) agreed with the supportive role of the nurse depicted by Nightingale, Henderson, Orem, Kinlein, and Abdellah, whilst for Travelbee (1971 p7) the consensus was with Peplau, in viewing nursing as:

> an interpersonal process whereby the professional nurse practitioner assists an individual, family, or community to prevent or cope with the experience of illness and suffering and, if necessary, to find meaning in these experiences.

The emphasis on interpersonal processes introduced a new way of defining nursing, allowing for people, who were in need of care, to be free to express their needs as unique humans.

King (1971 p22) continued the theme of nursing as being supportive in 'a process of action, reaction, interaction, and transaction'. For Roy (1976 p18) nursing activity was a matter of 'promoting man's adaptation in his physiological needs, his self concept, his role function and his interdependence relations during health and illness.' It is interesting to note the non-inclusive language used here, as a product of the time in which these words were written.

King and Roy shared the supportive function view of nursing espoused by previous authors, who were influenced by the biomedical model of health care of the empirico-analytical tradition, yet they were careful to acknowledge the uniqueness of the nurse-patient relationship in the nursing exchange. This unique relationship was named but undescribed, largely, in nursing literature until recent times, when interpretive ways of knowing were introduced into nursing literature. (Benner 1984, Benner & Wrubel 1989, Carper 1978, Chinn & Jacobs 1983, Dunlop 1986,1988, Gray & Pratt 1991, Kestenbaum 1982, Kretlow 1989–1990, Lawler 1991, Leininger 1985, Lumby 1991, McMahon & Pearson 1991, Munhall & Oiler 1986, Oiler 1982, 1986, Parker 1988, Parse 1985, Paterson & Zderad 1976, Pearson 1988b,1989, Taylor 1992a, Watson 1981, 1985).

Scholars in nursing have acknowledged the various ways of knowing, as evidenced by the history of epistemological enquiries in philosophy and other human sciences. This section will overview some literature relating to epistemological categorisations in nursing (Allen, Benner & Diekelmann 1986, Carper 1978, Chinn & Kramer 1991, Parse 1987).

Carper (1978) suggested four fundamental patterns of knowing in nursing: empirics, the science of nursing; aesthetics, the art of nursing; the component of personal knowledge in nursing; and ethics, the moral component. She acknowledged the contribution of all the patterns of knowing in increasing nurses' awareness of the diversity and complexity of nursing knowledge, emphasising that all forms of knowing have their place and none is mutually exclusive.

Chinn and Kramer (1991) extended the acknowledgement of equal importance and mutual inclusiveness of Carper's patterns of knowing in nursing, by emphasising the integrative aspects of knowing and describing the effects of 'patterns gone wild'. Respecting the context of the whole of knowing was acknowledged by Chinn and Kramer (1991 p15) in their warnings that:

> Empirics removed from the context of the whole of knowing produces control and manipulation...Ethics removed from the context of the whole of knowing produces rigid doctrine and insensitivity to the rights of others...Personal knowing removed from the context of the whole of knowing produces isolation and self distortion...Esthetics removed from the context of the whole of knowing produces prejudice, bigotry and lack of appreciation for meaning.

Allen, Benner and Diekelmann (1986 p23) supported 'a pluralistic vision of research methodology' by describing three paradigms for generating knowledge within nursing; the empirico-analytical paradigm, Heideggerian phenomenology, and critical social theory. These paradigms equate with Habermas' 'knowledge-constitutive interests,' by falling into technical, practical and emancipatory categorisations respectively. The technical interests include empirico-analytical ways of knowing, practical interests include interpretive ways of knowing and emancipatory interests include critical ways of knowing.

Parse (1987) categorised her own work into the Simultaneity paradigm, in contrast to the Totality paradigm, a natural or medical science approach to nursing she felt was reflected in the work of Peplau, Henderson, Hall, Orlando, Levine, Johnson, Roy, Orem and King. Parse (1987 p160) claimed that her work was a human science approach to nursing that viewed man as 'a unitary being in continuous mutual interrelationship with the environment.'

The epistemological categories suggested by Carper (1978) and reaffirmed by Chinn and Kramer (1991), can be subsumed into the paradigms described by Allen, Benner and Diekelmann (1986). The empirico-analytical paradigm includes empirics, Heideggerian phenomenology takes in personal knowing and aesthetics, and critical social science includes ethics and empirics. The Totality and

Simultaneity categories described by Parse reflect knowing in nursing in two main paradigms, which are suggestive of the empirico-analytical and phenomenological perspectives respectively.

Regardless of the ways in which nursing scholars present their epistemological categorisations, there is a consensus in recent writings (Allen, Benner & Diekelmann 1986, Carper 1978, Chinn & Kramer 1991, Parse 1987) that alternatives to positivistic understandings exist, and that nursing requires a mixture of epistemological approaches for finding meaning in nursing, and to portray the relative complexity and diversity of knowledge in a practice discipline. In contrast to this position, however, it should be noted that some scholars favour a careful selection of ways of knowing, a well quoted example being Beckstrand (1978a, 1978b, 1980), who argued against practice theory and claimed that nursing need only concern itself with the borrowed knowledge of science, and with knowledge of what is morally good, so that change, control, and ethical monitoring could be assured in and through nursing.

Knowing in nursing has been described by the ways in which it has been reflected in nursing definitions, and by the ways in which it has been categorised by nursing scholars. Epistemological enquiries about what counts as truth in nursing have been motivated by similar explorations in philosophy, which are perpetuated in nursing by the scholastic contributions of nursing authors.

Understanding how nurses regard Being and knowing in nursing not only gives nurses the means whereby they can find their personal and professional identities in nursing, it also contributes to defining nursing itself, through understanding the intricacies of interpersonal relationships in health care contexts. With these assumptions in mind, we return to the definition of nursing that I put forward previously, that nursing is whatever happens between nurses and patients in contexts of care, that is, nursing is whatever arises out of the necessity for nurses and patients to be together.

Knowledge that contributes towards the practice discipline of nursing

Disciplinary status is assigned to those areas of enquiry that can demonstrate that their knowledge constitutes something unique from other areas of knowledge interests. Time honoured disciplines include human sciences, such as philosophy and religion, and natural sciences, such as physics, chemistry, and biology. Relative to other disciplines, nursing is still in its academic infancy as it attempts to demonstrate its disciplinary status.

Being concerned with the development of professional knowledge and skills, nursing might more correctly be described as a
'practice discipline.' A practice discipline is one which prepares its
practitioners with knowledge for practice, as well as being concerned
with raising knowledge from the work experiences of its practitioners. The label of practice discipline has been central in the
debates about whether nursing has a body of knowledge which is
unique to its concerns, whether the core of nursing is the human
experiences of patients and nurses, and whether nursing can claim
that knowledge arises out the work of its practitioners.

The inability of nursing to define its nature and effects is related,
in part at least, to its inability to decide on the central locus of
nursing. Some nurses insist that they are doing nursing when they
are researching, teaching, or administering nursing; others claim
that nursing is what happens between nurses and patients in
contexts of nursing practice, and that the nurses who work in allied
areas of research, education and administration, and sundry other
nursing-oriented jobs, assist and support this important central
nurse-patient relationship.

When it is apparent that nurses are unsure about where nursing
occurs, under which circumstances, and with what effects, it
becomes plainer to see why they are also unsure about its disciplinary
status, and the kinds of knowledge that contribute to its unique
identity. In seeking to reach a consensus about what counts as truth
in nursing, questions need to be raised about the connections
between the nurse-patient relationship and the generation of an
unique body of knowledge in nursing. To date, the two main sides
of the disciplinary debate are that, as a practice discipline, nursing
borrows most of its knowledge from other disciplines, while the
opposing view asserts that there is theory inherent in everyday
nursing practice and, as such, the uniqueness of the nurse-patient
relationship provides sound knowledge for building up a disciplinary
base and growing theoretical framework.

The scholars who claim that nursing is a practice discipline argue
essentially that nursing is careful people-oriented work, of a health
related nature, which is energised by practice knowledge (Pearson
1988b, Smyth 1986, Tilden & Tilden 1985, Visintainer 1986).
For them, the combination of work for practical everyday purposes
with the knowledge that is needed for understanding the nature of
nursing gives nursing the label of a 'practice discipline.' In effect,
when nursing is referred to as a practice discipline, it conveys the
idea that nursing is concerned with the pursuit of knowledge for

practical purposes, thus the practice of nursing relates to professional issues of how, when, why, and with whom, nursing is done. In contrast, the opposing argument uses the label of practice discipline to argue the reverse, that the practice theory of nursing is borrowed from other disciplines and comprises scientific and moral knowledge mainly (Beckstrand 1978a, 1978b, 1980), and that, of itself, nursing has nothing or little to offer, as unique understandings, to itself, or to other established disciplines.

Nursing is about human experiences in health care contexts. The phenomena of nursing relate to the experiences of nurses and patients, in relation to the metaparadigm concepts of person, health, environment and nursing. Therefore, the discipline of nursing can be conveyed through theory, which depicts in words, the nature and effects of the phenomena constituting the concerns of nursing.

Donaldson and Crowley (1978) define a discipline as a 'unique perspective, a distinct way of viewing all phenomena, which ultimately defines the limits and nature of its enquiry.' Given this definition, and based on the premise that nursing is about 'hands-on' work with people, it would seem that a strong argument could be raised to contend that the central business of nursing is practice, and that the nature of nursing will be revealed by illuminating and articulating the nature and effects of nursing practice.

Johnson (1968 p3) defined borrowed theory as 'that knowledge which is developed in the main by other disciplines and is drawn upon by nursing.' Johnson agreed initially that nursing did not need to develop its own theory and, by thus doing, make claims to disciplinary status, although this stand was contradicted somewhat in her later work, when she noted that knowledge is not the possession of any one discipline, and that nursing needs to develop a unique theory of nursing that addresses issues of order, disorder, and control.

The tendency in nursing literature has been to polarise, and to keep distanced, nursing's professional and disciplinary endeavours. Such a polarisation finds its expression in arguments that the concerns of practice and theory are separate; that nursing is an applied science; that nurses with the mandate to research nursing should be kept apart from nursing practice; and that practice informs practitioners, but not the disciplinary content of nursing (Beckstrand 1978a, 1978b, Donaldson & Crowley 1978, Gortner 1983).

A different perspective, however, claims that theory and practice can be considered as mutually synergistic (Pearson 1988b); that nursing is known in a variety of ways (Carper 1978); that nurses, who are practitioners, can be theorisers of their own work (Smyth

LOTHIAN COLLEGE OF HEALTH STUDIES LIBRARY

d that the practice of nursing can inform the discipline of by virtue of its nature and location as the central business g (Tilden & Tilden 1985, Visintainer 1986). Hence, rather than continuing to see professional work and disciplinary theory as being two separate dimensions in nursing, an alternate view would be to see them as creating a dialogue with one another, to reconcile their apparent contradictions (Moccia 1986).

The tendency to label nursing as an 'applied science', based on the contributions other disciplines make to nursing, is shared by some nurses, who agree with Beckstrand (1978a, 1978b) that all knowledge necessary for nursing is borrowed, leaving nursing without its own unique identity and practice theory. Counter to this view is the claim that nursing is known in a variety of ways (Carper 1978) and that the generation of knowledge from borrowed as well as original sources in the practice of nursing, creates the substance of a practice discipline (Pearson 1988b).

The polarised positions of professional and disciplinary concerns have been maintained by nurses, who work with the assumption that the people best able to research nursing are those nurses who are able to remain aloof from the nurses who 'roll up their sleeves' in the daily grind of practice (Donaldson & Crowley 1978). Such a stance sets theoretical pursuits operationalised in research projects as separate and superior. Research activities are thereby assigned to those nurses who are seen as being somehow intellectually superior to those nurses who are entrusted with the everyday care of people. A contrasting view would be that professional and disciplinary issues can create a dialogue between practice and theory, when nurses, who are practitioners, are encouraged to become theorisers of their own work (Smyth 1986).

Arguing that science seeks universal truths and that practical knowledge and clinical wisdom in practice cannot move from the particular, Gortner (1983a, 1983b) contended that practice informs practitioners on local levels, but that it cannot inform the disciplinary content of nursing in general. This view places immense faith in the tenets of scientific knowledge or empirics, whilst under-estimating the equal contributions made to nursing theories by aesthetics, personal knowledge and ethical patterns of knowing (Carper 1978, Chinn & Kramer 1991).

Keeping theory away from practice settings, from fear of tainting the purity of conceptual constructions performed by nurse academics, with the everyday work concerns of nursing performed by clinical nurses (Gortner 1983a, 1983b), has controlled interaction and understanding between communities of nurses. Nurses have tended to see the everyday labour of nursing as something less worthy than the hallowed work of nurse researchers and academics. Nurses have steered their courses away from the bedside, community-side, and homeside practice of nursing, to employment in administrative and academic areas, believing that the prestige of these positions elevated them above the morass of daily nursing practice.

The practice arenas of nursing and the established theory-producing areas of other nursing-related contexts need not be kept apart. Permitted a continuing dialogue, professional issues of practice and disciplinary concerns of theory could be mutually synergistic. The dialogue could be between equal partners, if one agrees with Pearson (1988b) that nursing practice is 'a sophisticated intellectual pursuit, which incorporates a variety of patterns of knowing.' When the two meet and collaborate with each other to sort out their similarities and inconsistencies, the synergistic effect could begin to illuminate and interpret the complexities of nursing itself.

The tensions may be reconciled by the recognition that practice can inform the discipline of nursing, by virtue of its nature and location as the central business of nursing (Tilden & Tilden 1985, Visintainer 1986). The nature of nursing is to nurse; it is what practitioners do. To impose theories on practice generated away from the context of practice is tantamount to a penguin telling airborne birds how to fly. Practitioners know themselves and they can be encouraged to find ways to uncover and express the sophisticated knowledge they embody in their day to day nursing interactions (Smyth 1986, Street 1990, 1991, Taylor 1990).

It can be seen, therefore, that when the so-called opposing views of professional and disciplinary concerns are brought together, that the dialogue can be exceedingly valuable to the profession and the discipline of nursing. The separation of the two has been maintained, much as the separation of practice and theory has been perpetuated, by creating diametrically opposed identities, which serve to rob each of the value of the other. Rather than deplete the generative sources of each other by separation, a reconciliation of the perspectives in terms of a critique of their similarities and differences, can fortify nursing as a practice discipline.

The nature and effects of the nurse-patient relationship

Humanistic qualities in the nurse-patient relationship have been addressed in the literature, as the themes of authenticity, concern and presencing. Jourard (1971 p182) claimed that 'people squelch their real selves, because they have learned to fear the consequences of authentic being.' He was suspicious particularly of the 'nurse's bedside manner,' as a facade to shield her or him from the vulnerability inherent in her or his own humanness. He concluded that a nurse who was unwilling to be authentic in her or his self-disclosures, was in fact blocking the patient's chances for self-disclosure and authenticity.

Derived from existential phenomenology, the notion of authenticity has been taken up by nursing scholars (Benner 1984, Benner & Wrubel 1989, Parse 1987), who have explored some possibilities for choices in nursing practice, as nurses decide courses of action in their day to day work.

Benner and Wrubel (1989 p47) used the word 'concern' in the Heideggerian sense, to mean something more than commitment. Heidegger (1962 trans. p158-159) gave two examples of concern: first, the kind of solicitude that leaps in and 'takes over for the Other that with which he is to concern himself'; and second, the kind of solicitude that 'leaps ahead' of the Other, 'not in order to take away his (or her) "care" but rather to give it back to him (or her) authentically.' Using the phenomenological concept of concern to describe person and interpersonal relationships as things that really matter, Benner and Wrubel (1989 p49) point out that although the first kind of concern is necessary when patients are unable to cope by themselves, the second kind of solicitude 'is a form of advocacy and facilitation. It empowers the Other to be what he or she wants to be, and this is the ultimate goal in nursing care relationships.'

The Heideggerian concept of presencing (Heidegger 1962 trans.) has been used to describe the availability of the nurse to understand the patient, by a process of human relating. As Benner and Wrubel (1989 p13) explain 'the ability to presence oneself, to be with the patient in a way that acknowledges your shared humanity, is the base of much of nursing as a caring practice.' This statement poses a different view from the professional ethic of distancing and aloofness, in which professionals avoid the risks of personal involvement, by hiding in their 'character armour' and acting out a repertoire of behaviours consistent with the 'professional manner' (Jourard 1971).

Campbell (1985) described nursing as skilled companionship that entails sharing freely and not imposing, thus allowing others to make their own life journey. He conceptualised nursing as involving a bodily presence, in sensing need and accomodating idiosyncrasies (sensitivity); in helping onwards to recovery or death (encouraging); in risking to be with, staying with the difficult point (being with); and in allowing the other to go on alone (limitation). Thus, he saw nursing as a love-companionship relationship.

Love-companionship in nursing involving sensitivity, being with, and allowing for limitation of the caring role, is therapeutic in nature and outcome. The word therapeutic is derived from the Greek *therapeutikos* from therapeue in meaning to minister to (Collins English Dictionary 1986). In health care, therapeutics has taken on a disease-curing connotation traditionally, leaving curing to doctors, and caring to nurses. Therapeutic counselling has also been connected with psychoanalytic approaches, which suggest that counsellors maintain their distance in their professional relationships.

Therapeutics and therapy are taking on new connotations in nursing. The claim has been made that nursing is both 'carative' and curative (Benner & Wrubel 1989, Kitson 1984, Pearson,1988c) and that care is the essence of nursing (Leininger 1985, Watson 1985). Although caring is the most obvious and regularly described attribute of nursing, they argue that it is not the sole mission of nursing. The therapeutic potential of nursing is related to the science of nursing and to the artistry with which nursing care is given.

Rather than seeing therapeutics as the sole province of doctors, or regarding therapy as occurring in distanced professional relationships, nurses are claiming the worth of their presence, and they are beginning to explore the nature and effects of therapeutic relationships in nursing. First introduced into the literature by Peplau (1952), who described nursing as a therapeutic relationship, nursing scholars (Pearson 1988c, McMahon & Pearson 1991) are beginning to explore the therapeutic potential of nursing, in terms of its healing possibilities. Claims for therapeutic effects in nursing have arisen from authors' interpretations of the nature of the nurse-patient relationship. Pearson (1988c p12) claims that exploration of therapeutic approaches in nursing care can get at the heart of practice, that is, into the nurse-patient relationship, when professional detachment is abandoned in favour of 'closeness between nurse and patient, the idea of partnership, and the development of empathy in nursing.' The effect of this closeness is considered to be healing in nature, as a form of therapeutic nursing.

Meutzel (in Pearson 1988c p89) supported the contention that nursing is a 'therapy in itself,' confirming that 'the power of nursing to promote healing lies...in this therapeutic relationship,' that endorses 'the therapeutic use of self' and characterises the nurse-patient relationship with partnership, intimacy and reciprocity.

In contrast to nursing as therapy, Swaffield (1988) gave an example of 'anti-therapy', in which a nurse was not in tune with the patient, batting off his need to express his fears with inappropriate comments, which stifled effective communication, saving the nurse from further involvement with the patient. The conditions necessary for therapeutic interactions were described by a primary nurse, who explained that:

[y]ou have to remove your ego, and get into the patient's frame of reference. Some people are naturals at it, but everyone can learn to do it. Only then does the contact become therapeutic. Of course you can't be totally tuned into somebody else all the time. It's a bit like therapeutic touch—it has to be turned on. The difference then, is between being efficient and being switched on. It means listening and befriending, as well as doing. It means holding back self-protecting 'nursey' instincts and substituting more human ones. It even means handling responsibility, and problems back to the patients (p31).

The therapeutic nature of nursing is related to the healing effects of nurses and patients interacting as humans together. Something more than nurses' knowledge and skills accounts for the healing effects, because the therapeutic effects are reciprocated between nurses and patients, that is, nurses and patients alike can experience the various benefits of their relationship. There is something about the humanness of both parties, and the ways in which they combine together in the relatively strange contexts of health care facilities, that holds within it the reasons for therapeutic effects in nursing. Central to this assumption is my thesis about the phenomenon of ordinariness in nursing, that is, the sense of shared affinity nurses and patients have as humans creates for them a bond which transcends their apparent differences as nurses and patients. It is my claim that it is ordinariness in nursing, that sense of shared affinity nurses and patients have for one another as humans, that accounts, at least in part, for the caring and curing that occurs when nurses and patients relate to one another as humans in health care contexts.

Nurses do clinical work and it is through this work that the quality of 'being with' is expressed. Doing is related to being, in that nurses and patients express their being together through the vehicle of 'doing for', and 'being done to, and with'. Nurses become very skilled at doing things; 'doing for' is how they reflect their knowledge and skills and deliver nursing care. 'Doing for' is related to 'being with,' when nurses attend to the quality of the nurse-patient relationship through which patients' goals are negotiated, set and accomplished.

McPherson (1987) connected nurses' 'doing for' to the author's lived experience of diabetes mellitus. The author, who is a nurse, recounted her experience of being in hospital to clarify some concepts of phenomenology and hermeneutics. Of particular interest in her account was how the doing of nursing is connected to the 'being' of a patient.

Doing and being relate to the subject of therapeutic nursing. Nurses are notorious 'doers,' and nursing care plans document, to some extent, the quantity and quality of their nursing actions. Tasks directed towards patients' physiological outcomes are well known to nurses. Lists of duties, such as four hourly observations, changes of patients' positions in bed, fluid balance monitoring, dressing changes, and so on, are aimed at restoring, supporting, and maintaining, patients' physiological processes. All of these tasks are necessary, but they reflect biomedical imperatives mainly, rather than modes of caring that show creative healing imagination.

Nurses are beginning to consider the use of complementary therapies in their repertoire of nursing care skills. Imagine a nursing care plan, for instance, that lists, along with the procedural tasks that check and maintain physiologic functions, other creative alternatives for patients, matched to their experiences of illness, such as aromatherapy, massage, reminiscence sessions, singalongs, creative writing, and so on. Rather than being used solely as therapies in themselves, these modalities, and many more (Unit NPR 305 Bibliography 1993), may be used as vehicles for being with patients, for creating time and space in which therapeutic nursing can be potentiated.

One vehicle for communication between nurses and patients is that of touch (Tutton 1991). Touch is integral to nursing care and in its various forms it can mean different things to patients. Touch and touching can facilitate human connections. It is important to remember that complementary therapies used in nursing care are vehicles for therapeutic encounters; they do not replace the human connection within the situation. If these complementary therapies become the latest craze for quick fix solutions to nursing care problems, in time they may become as routinised as many other nursing tasks that direct the nurse's attention to the 'doing for' and away from the 'being with.'

Therapeutic nursing relates to the quality of the nurse-patient relationship and how this relationship mobilises healing responses in individuals. Valuing therapeutic nursing is valuing the nurse-patient relationship, as a potentiating force in health care.

The idea that nurses are healers may be new to some people. Generally speaking, the nursing literature has supported nurses' views of themselves, as masked carers, performing within the safety of their professional roles. The indeterminacy of their clinical lives, and a host of other constraints operating on them within their particular health care cultures, have moulded nurses' approaches to nursing care, and dictated their ways of being and knowing whenever they have interacted with patients, and the patients' families and friends.

Essentially, nurses have been typified in nursing literature as dispensers of nursing care, within the authority of their professional roles. Nurses have been depicted as supporting the curative properties of Nature (Henderson 1966, Nightingale 1859), as facilitators of patients' stimulus-response mechanisms (Johnson 1980, Orlando 1961, Peplau 1952, Roy 1976) and as health professionals, who direct patients towards goal attainment (Abdellah et al 1960, Hall 1964, King 1971 1981, Neuman 1989,Orem 1985, Wiedenbach 1964).

What has been less apparent in nursing practice and its supporting literature, has been permission for nurses to transcend the confines of their role responsibilities and institutional expectations, to revisit their own humanity within themselves, so that it can be freed to surface in day to day nursing care. The effects of being human in professional contexts are related to therapeutic outcomes. Nurses become therapists and nursing becomes therapy, when nurses' knowledge and skills are shared in human ways, that are recognised and appreciated as such by the people for whom they care.

An introduction to the research

It seems that human life is full of diversity and activity. People vary according to their their race, colour, creed, and may other variables such as their age, gender, culture, education and social position and more, and the fullness and untapped potential of the material world allows for seemingly endless human activity. As unique individuals, we go about our everyday lives experiencing this variety in human life by interacting with the people and things around us. It is as if we exist as single units of humanity, who bump occasionally up against one another in the pursuit of finding some meaning in our humanness. Our uniqueness as individuals and our bodily parameters tend to separate us from other people around us, making us feel alone ultimately.

Even though human life may be full of diversity and activity, the one thing which connects all human beings together regardless of their race, colour, creed or any other differentiating category we might choose to name, is their shared sense of what it means to be a human being. In my research, I interacted with nurses and patients and I found that their shared sense of humanity made them as one in the context of nursing care. As a general group, these people had certain shared human qualities that had enhancing effects on their individual existences as nurses and patients.

The nurses and patients in the research recognised and respected each other as human beings and although they were aware of their differences, in terms of living their separate experiences of 'being a nurse' and 'being a patient,' they nevertheless were as one in the ordinariness of their humanity. The shared sense of being human between nurses and patients made them as one in their humanness and created a special place, in which the relative strangeness of the experience of being in a health care setting could be made familiar and manageable.

How the idea for the research was generated

The idea of researching the phenomenon of ordinariness in nursing originated from discussions with Professor Alan Pearson, a nurse, who made some clinical observations in his own nursing practice that, when he joked and generally took time to interact on an ordinary human level with patients, the experience of nursing was enhanced for his patients and himself (1988a).

In some previous research into nursing practice (Taylor 1988), I found that when I asked women in a postnatal ward to describe the midwives who were most effective in caring for them, they described those midwives who were 'just themselves.' The mothers differentiated carefully between those midwives who they perceived as 'professional' in a detached way, and the midwives who they perceived as ordinary human beings in spite of their clinical effectiveness.

The background to the research, therefore, included an interest in the phenomenon springing from an original idea as expressed by Pearson (1988a) and the results of my own research and clinical experience.

What the research hoped to achieve

Essentially, the research wanted to explore nurse-patient relationships, so that the nature and effects of ordinariness could be manifested clearly, to see whether or not it enhanced nursing encounters. I proposed the research in the hope of raising some possibilities for more effective nursing practice, and in so doing to add to that body of knowledge that comprises the practice discipline of nursing.

I decided that a phenomenological approach would be a useful way of exploring the phenomenon of ordinariness. Using the experiences and language of some nurses and patients involved in everyday nursing encounters, the phenomenon expressed the potential of everyday human qualities and activities in nursing. A fuller explanation of phenomenology and the reasons for its selection as a guide for undertaking this research, will be given later in Chapter 2.

Early thoughts about ordinariness in nursing

The Oxford Dictionary records the historical meanings of the word 'ordinary.' In relation to language, ordinary is 'the most commonly found or attested,' and in relation to people, ordinary is 'typical of a particular group, average...' The sense of ordinary, for both language and people, is that of shared qualities. Whatever the unique characteristics of each individual, people are bonded by their ordinary status of humanity, bearing with it certain qualities that are grouped as typical, and these are vital for understanding the ways in which they communicate with one another and make meaning of their existence together.

Although it was acknowledged that 'ordinariness' would assume its own identity through the research process, I decided to review some literature to have a glimpse at what ordinariness might be. My rationale for undertaking a literature review at this stage was related to a methodological assumption underlying the method I used that, by virtue of my Being-in-the-world and my inextricability with other humans and human events, my subjective nature as a person afforded me some knowledge of human existence; so it was pointless of me to pretend that I had no presuppositions of the phenomenon, or that things I learned along the way would not be taken into account in the final analysis.

I began with an indistinct idea of what ordinariness might be, thinking it to be something like 'being yourself,' or 'being human.' I reviewed some literature relating to natural therapies and indigenous therapists, in the hope that I might arrive at some characteristics of people, suggestive of those persons who are engaged in natural caring and curing processes. I also reviewed some contemporary and nursing literature relating, more specifically, to ordinariness.

Natural therapies and indigenous therapists

The literature relating to natural therapies dealt with the types of therapies, the critique of the therapies in relation to their superstitious or scientific content, the cultural patterns of acceptance of the therapies, the dilemmas of practitioners who work on the interface of specific cultural acceptance of therapies, and the future in relation to the perspectives of healing.

There are many alternative therapies available to people that provide a contrast to Western medicine and ways of managing illness from a biomedical perspective in the 20th century. The vast range of therapies available claim some measure of success, when used as intended (Forbes 1985, Author unknown 1988). The most commonly used therapies centre on the use of herbs. (Cooper 1984, Potterton 1983). Interestingly, nurses have successfully used a wide range of natural therapies in their work (Cate 1986, Dobbs 1985, Hillman 1986a 1986b, O'Grady 1989, Turton 1986, Weaver 1985, Westwood 1986).

Critiques of alternative therapies have often been in relation to their superstitious content. (Boxall 1988, Dring 1985, Motlana 1988, Rosser 1982). In contrast to these positions, the power of superstition has been acclaimed (Searle 1980, Warner 1977, Wooding 1983). Carstairs (1977 p337) explained that what these traditional helpers give to their clients—and also to the 'significant others' in their immediate family circle—is a powerful infusion of confidence that the outcome will be alright, provided they perform the prescribed rituals.

The cultural patterns of acceptance of therapies varies according to the beliefs and practices of the people concerned. In a study in the West Indies, Aho and Minott (1977) found that local people use Creole cures mostly and that they have unfavourable attitudes towards 'doctor medicine'. Here, Creole cures have persisted because the local people believe they work. Hall and Bourne (1973 p139) found that the practices of root doctors, faith healers, magic vendors, and neighbourhood prophets continued to flourish, based on the popularity of these healers and their 'ability to provide practical advice on the everyday problems, that confront their largely poverty stricken and deprived' clients.

Tripp-Reimer (1983) reported on the folk healing practice (matiasma) among a population of urban Greek immigrants in Ohio and found that they retained their ethnomedical beliefs and practices, because they were convinced of the validity of the 'evil eye' as causation of disease. Tripp-Reimer advocated that these beliefs should be respected by nurses working with these people. Flanagin (1989) reported that spirits and traditional medicine coexist in Liberia, with most faith being placed in the former. Green (1985 p283) advocated that, in Swaziland, 'health education strategy must begin with an acknowledgement that traditional medical beliefs and practices are unusually tenacious...'

The power of folk beliefs and the need to work in relation to them, has been acknowledged in Nigeria (Asuni 1979, Jegede, Williams & Sijuwola 1985, Odebiyi & Togonu-Bickersteth 1987). Awareness of all, and integration of some, accepted folk health practices has been suggested by some nurses (Capers 1985, Glittenberg 1974, Olsson 1989, Rosenblum 1980). The acceptance or rejection of some folk remedies was judged according to the empirical validity of each therapy, as measured primarily by Western standards.

The literature highlighted the dilemmas experienced by practitioners, who work on the interface of folk and scientific therapies (Barbee 1986, Gregory & Stewart 1987, Lee 1986, Mackenzie 1987, Ranin 1978). The assumption seems to be that there is a dichotomy between folk and professional health practice; however, Robertson (1987b) found that health professionals held some beliefs that could be considered folk health beliefs and that they integrated scientific and folk beliefs in their practices. Swanwick (1986) and Goldstein (undated) suggested ways in which alternative medicine could be integrated into current health care.

Darbyshire (1985) and Gartrell (1987) interpreted the tension between folk and scientific therapies as gender-related. Darbyshire (1985 p44) contended that:

> [f]or the aspiring male medical profession, the wise woman-healer posed a threat not only to their male control of healing but also to the exclusiveness of the profession, concerned as it was with the jealous guarding of health and illness knowledge.

In support of Darbyshire, Gartrell (1987 p23) also claimed that:

> [r]esearch interests traditionally have been focussed on the development of the medical profession, institutions, and scientific breakthroughs rather than on the experiences of ordinary people. And when women were mentioned at all, sometimes the view was disparaging.

Kleinman (1977) acknowledged the value of folk beliefs and suggested there was a need for interdisciplinary research into explaining the efficacy of indigenous therapies. A common theme in the literature was the future, in relation to the perspectives of healing. Kleinman (1978a, 1978b, in Anderson 1987) described three structural domains of health care in society; professional, popular and folk. 'Professional' represented Western medicine with its physicians, nurses, and other health professionals; 'popular' represented family and community treatment; and 'folk' referred to non-professional healing specialists. Anderson (1987) supported 'a nurse-patient negotiation model' which delivered 'culturally sensitive care,' especially in the light of the greater percentage of treatment falling within the non-professional areas.

Lamb (1987) and Bulbrook (1984) attested to the value of the use of alternative approaches to cater for the future. Bulbrook (1984 p27) contrasted the two health care systems thus:

[in one] the patient is considered autonomous and the professional is viewed as the professional partner, whereas [in the other] the medical paradigm views the professional as an authority figure, the patient as dependent and the disease or disability is considered as a thing, as an entity.

Eisenberg (1977 p9) called for a reintegration of 'scientific and social concepts of disease and illness as a basis for a functional system of medical research and care.' The predictions for the future were essentially optimistic if there could be an integration of approaches which assisted in manifesting the reality of holistic care. The reality relied heavily on a continuing critique of the philosophy and consequences of Cartesian dualism and a return to natural approaches centred on humanistic concerns.

The literature relating to natural therapies showed that their perpetuation is due to the trust held in them by the therapists and clients who use them. People choose the traditional approaches over biomedical care, because they believe natural therapies are therapeutic and that they, as individuals, have some control in their treatment. For these people, the return to traditional health care was tantamount to a return to holism, rejecting the reductionism of biomedicine and its proponents.

The intention in searching the literature relating to indigenous therapists and traditional healers, was to ascertain whether there were any human qualities, which set these people apart as part of their ordinary ways of being. I was motivated to find out whether, indeed, there was some connection between their everyday qualities as humans and their effectiveness.

Indigenous therapists are people, who are sanctioned by a particular culture or subculture to do therapeutic, interpersonal work, even though they have not been trained to do so by acceptable Western professional standards. The need for indigenous therapists is greater in settings where the health needs of the population exceed the ability of professionals to manage adequately. The literature tended to report experiences in psychiatric, geriatric and hospice areas.

Torrey (1969 p365) found that possible therapeutic effects of indigenous therapists were due to their qualities of 'accurate empathy, nonpossessive warmth, and genuineness' and concluded that indigenous therapists are often effective in producing positive therapeutic changes by understanding the philosophy of the people and by knowing how to 'placate the troubled by plausible interpretation of their troubles.'

Stevenson and Viney (1973) found that nonprofessionals enjoyed some measure of success with psychotic patients, even though the patients were deemed to be hopeless, the difficulties of establishing a meaningful dialogue were considered to be great, and the ward staff was noticeably unco-operative.

Rosenbaum (in Scott Verinis 1970) 'explained the therapeutic success of the untrained personnel in terms of eagerness, enthusiasm, and general unawareness of the implicit principle that chronic patients cannot be helped.' This was is in contrast with the pessimism of professional staff, whose defeatism limited their therapeutic effectiveness. Scott Verinis (1970) found gains in the treatment group and in tentatively attributing it to the nonprofessionals, questioned whether 'warm, sympathetic, continuing, and enthusiastic interest that is hypothesized to be so therapeutic, could be used by others.'

Authors (Carstairs 1977, Sanda 1978) attested to the magical qualities of the indigenous therapist and described the differences between the magical ways of knowing exemplified by the traditional healer and scientific ways of knowing enacted in Western medicine.

In looking at the literature on traditional healers, it was evident that they were aware of the total social context in which they worked and lived, and that their approaches took these considerations into account. A non-professional approach to caring was practised, in that the indigenous therapist was not constrained by stereotypes and the pessimism of professional approaches, being free to interact with clients in a natural and context-specific way. The literature informed the research potentially, by suggesting some qualities and conditions of therapeutic ordinariness, which may become evident and be shown as therapeutic in nursing encounters.

Ordinariness

Although the phenomenon of ordinariness, per se, has not been described widely in the literature, other synonyms have been used to depict themes surrounding everyday interpersonal interactions. In acknowledging the importance of ordinary life, Goffman (1974) likened day to day life to performances of actors on a stage and claimed that actors have some protection against daily contingencies, unlike ordinary life in which people play out each moment as it comes.

Day to day interactions may become so well understood, that co-operation is achieved through internalising elements of the world, through symbolic thought, so that understandings are not necessarily articulated but remain integral to the fabric of social interactions. Douglas (1974 p27) described his interpretations of everyday life, that:

> most important, human beings cannot live without cooperating with other human beings, and human thought, which is essentially symbolic thought, cannot exist without a high degree of this cooperation from our earliest days...

The shareability of knowledge rests on the familiarity of people with one another in their unique contexts. For people involved in practical thinking, knowledge about the everyday world becomes so taken for granted that it is not relayed explicitly, but understood implicitly. The ordinary commonsense knowledge is not unimportant, rather it becomes part of the nature of the social group to the extent that it becomes invisible. In this view, Douglas (1974 p27) claimed that all human knowledge is necessarily shared knowledge, secrets excepting, thus we have commonsense knowledge that is shared. He explained:

> [t]his shareability of knowledge is so fundamental to doing practical thinking that it comes to be taken for granted for all 'competent' or 'ordinary' members of any social group. Indeed, the forms of knowledge most take for granted in any group come to be seen as absolute—as independent of the knowing minds, as out there.

Malone and Malone (1987) used the word ordinariness in relation to interpersonal relationships. They perceived that people who accepted and nurtured their ordinariness were reacting naturally to life events. They explained that in the attempt to do what we think we should do, rather than what we would like to do, we think that we have to be special; so we strive to please others and risk the effects of high stress rates, rather than simply being ordinary, which is what we are, and how we are meant to be, as humans.

In explicating their view of ordinariness, Malone and Malone (1987) claimed ordinariness means to behave outwards from ourselves, and not in terms of what is outside us. They explained that no-one wants to be thought of as common, average or ordinary, thus they attempt to be special and create a facade which they think portrays the self in a good light. They explained that the result of this action is that people fill their lives with stress trying to be special, because it takes a lot of energy to act against one's ordinary behaviour. They suggested that 'at some point we go forward to be what we ordinarily are' and that 'this does not mean not to pursue all that we can be. It means that we must pursue it without the loss of what we are' (p137). Ordinariness was portrayed as a powerful and an appropriate way of being. Quoting George Eliot (in Malone & Malone 1987 p136) they suggested that:

> [i]f we had a keen vision of all that is ordinary in human life, it would be like hearing the grass grow or the squirrel's heart beat, and we should die of the roar which is the other side of silence. Ordinariness, indeed, has the power, it is what is.

This view was also forwarded by Moore (1989), who provided a spiritual perspective of living the ordinary life by suggesting that, as humans, our nature is love and that love is absolutely ordinary. She was careful to point out that she did not use the word ordinary to mean mediocrity, rather she used it in the sense of simple, as in uncomplicated. She explained that:

> [o]rdinary is the answer. To be 'simple' in the moment will give you a sense of how you can just let go. In the letting go, your bound-up energy is released. The energy that is left can be used in a more creative way...By allowing yourself to experience the incredible wonder of the ordinary, you will create a space that allows other people to also be who they are (p104).

Everyday sharing and feeling has been described. Fook (1988) described the concept of social empathy, in which a therapist is able to understand the situation of a client. I imagined that something of this kind of empathy might be evident in ordinariness in nursing; however, in contrast to the relatively contrived therapist-client situation, the empathy possible through ordinariness seems to transcend a merely professional level, to one which is that of genuine intersubjective closeness.

Ordinariness might also have to do with being so 'at home' in a context, that it is possible to let go of some of the behaviours which normally protect the individual from personal vulnerability. Goffman (1961) described the sociological concept of role distancing, in which the person assumed a disdainful relation to a usual role. Role distancing occurred in contextually appropriate interactions, having a naturalness and humour about it which had meaning for the people in that encounter.

The review of the literature showed that ordinariness is not, as might be first thought, a phenomenon to be dismissed as inconsequential to everyday life, but that it is the very nature of who people are as humans, and how they relate to one another in day to day interpersonal interactions. In turning around the popular notions of the word 'ordinary,' as something which is unremarkable, these writers seemed to attest to the value of ordinariness as a phenomenon of everyday life which emphasised, rather than trivialised, the essential nature of humans in their day to day worlds.

Ordinariness in nursing

Although ordinariness, per se, has not been addressed in nursing literature, nurses have written about the shared humanity of the nurse-patient relationship. The work of these authors has been described previously.

Nursing practice reflects the ways nurses and patients experience the nurse-patient relationship, which is inextricably bound to the humanness of the people. Speaking at a nurse graduation ceremony, Pearson (1988a) said:

> [a]lthough I passionately believe that nursing, and therefore helping, must draw on knowledge, understandings and insights which are part of good quality professional education, I also believe that it is important to marry this with the ordinariness of being a human being...Most of us are engaged in the process of helping people every day, often without any conscious awareness of 'being helpful.' The foundation of genuine helping lies in being ordinary. Nothing special. We can offer ourselves, neither more nor less, to others—we have in fact nothing else to give. Anything more is conceit, anything less is robbing those in distress.

Accounts have been given, by nurses and patients, of what it means to exist in the world of nursing. Gino (1985 p30) described her freedom to be herself as a nurse interacting with other human beings.

> It was the one place I could be totally me. The place I could be as smart, as kind, as giving, and as real as I was capable of being. My patients and I had an understanding past words; we needed each other; we healed each other; and neither of us judged the other. There was no mask, no preference, we were just human beings who because of circumstances had to learn to trust each other and so were allowed to really touch each other.

Helman (1986) told the story of the illness of her husband, a cancer surgeon, who died of cancer. He recorded on audiotapes his reactions to his dying. He emphasised the need for basic confidence, a sense of hope, concern, compassion and humility from the people around him; all of which seem to be fairly ordinary human qualities. Nurses who reflect their ordinary humanness retain who they are and how they are, in spite of temptations to hide inside their 'character armour' (Jourard 1971). Being human is being ordinary; we laugh and we cry, we intellectualise and we become downright irrational. It may be possible that, in becoming sophisticated in nursing skills and knowledge, nurses may have lost sight of their essential nature as people. 'One of the difficulties with being sophisticated is a negation of the natural...they do not have to be separate' (Moore 1986 p169).

I was able to create a firmer conceptual framework for the research, following my review of literature. In recognition of the inductive, exploratory nature of phenomenological research and my awareness of some of my own preconceptions, it seemed possible that ordinariness might include notions of nurses and patients within caring relationships, creating meaning for themselves, and for the practice discipline of nursing.

Some notions incorporating the conceptual framework were: being oneself in a strange situation (Malone & Malone 1987, Moore 1989, Pearson 1988a, Taylor 1988); accurate empathy, nonpossessive warmth, and genuineness (Torrey 1969); authenticity, concern and presencing (Heidegger 1962 trans.) and nursing as a therapeutic relationship (McMahon & Pearson 1991, Pearson 1988c, Peplau 1952); all of which had the potential of creating meaning for the nurse and patient and for the practice discipline of nursing.

The setting for the research

The further away from home people go, the further they are separated from the familiarity of their own place of existence, and their daily practices of living. When people become patients they may need to go away from their homes into artificial, health care settings and it is reasonable to imagine that this relocation may well result in a variety of negative feelings by patients, and for those people to whom they matter.

Nurses work in a variety of settings ranging from the patients' own homes to more foreign contexts, such as community centres and hospital wards. When nurses go into homes in their professional capacities, they are entering patients' private existences, much as any other person would who enters their home as a guest. Clinical settings in community and hospital buildings present a different situation to that experienced in private homes. Patients leave home to attend clinical settings and nurses are waiting there to meet and care for them.

When patients and nurses meet in the shared space of community offices or hospital wards, the environment may be a far cry from the familiarity of their homes and this may well affect the nature of how they communicate there. Clinical settings do not always lend themselves well to people's needs, indeed it may be argued that they are set up more for organisational convenience, than for people's benefits.

In the research project, which is the focus of this book, the health care context was a Professorial Nursing Unit (PNU), which was established as a separate nursing area within a traditional hospital organisation. The PNU was in a large acute care hospital in Victoria, Australia. It was based on the Burford and Oxford Nursing Development Units, which were set up in the United Kingdom by Alan Pearson, who was the foundation Professor of the PNU in this research.

People admitted into nursing beds in these units are deemed to require nursing care as their main health need, thus the PNU structures and practices support therapeutic care organised on primary nursing. Patient care is organised and directed by nurses and the structure and processes of the units are geared towards making the environment more homely, so that patients can feel as comfortable as possible. Nurses do not wear uniforms and patients are encouraged to dress in day clothes and to remain as close as possible to their usual activities of daily living.

In this research, primary nursing was the system of nursing care delivery chosen in the Professorial Nursing Unit, because the staff 'believe that the structure of primary nursing promotes individualised care and greater continuity of care' (Workshop report document 1989 p16). There were two Primary Nurses, who led their respective nursing teams. Nurses in the PNU were allocated periodically to a different team and therefore experienced a different mix of leadership style, team composition and patient case load.

The PNU was set up with the intention of transcending, as far as possible, the institutional constraints of the hospital environment. On a practical level, this includes a tea room and games area for patients, and freer rules for patient mobility within and outside the unit. The unit gives approval to first name bases between staff and patients, and it consents explicitly to nurses and patients spending time together as people. Involvement of family and friends in the person's hospitalisation is encouraged, and interpersonal relationships are emphasised as being integral to therapeutic outcomes in nursing care.

Based in part on the experience of the Loeb Centre in New York, which was established by Lydia Hall, nursing development units have been pioneered in Great Britain by Alan Pearson (1983a, 1983b, 1984a, 1984b, 1985a, 1985b, 1985c, 1985d) and are presently reproducing at a rapid rate throughout that nation. Nursing development units have nursing care as their central concern and use the practice of therapeutic nursing (Pearson 1988c, 1988f, 1988h, 1990a, 1990b) for the outcomes of positive patient outcome experiences, high quality assurance scores and low running costs. The experience of the Burford (Pearson 1984c, 1985a, 1985b) and Oxford Nursing Development Units (Pearson 1988d, 1988e, 1988f, Pearson, Durand & Punton 1988a, 1988b, 1989) showed these benefits of using care giving 'based on therapeutic relationships and the therapeutic use of touch and massage' (Pearson 1988c p125).

Some assumptions and key terms explained

I have not given explanations of medical and nursing terms that I have used in this book, because I imagine that many of the readers will be health professionals. If professional familiarity with the words is not the case for you, they can be located in a medical or nursing dictionary.

In many cases, I have reserved the right to describe myself as a person, by referring to myself as 'I' instead of 'the researcher.' This is in acknowledgement of the nature of interpretive research and in deep respect for my personal encounters with the people in this research.

In sections of this book in which parts of conversations are relayed, some extra words are supplied in brackets, to enhance the reader's comprehension of the context and to assist the flow of grammar.

The main terms central to understanding this book are supplied below in alphabetical order:

Actualities. The parts that show the actual nature of the thing (phenomenon) itself, its 'Dasein,' or 'There-Being.'

Aspects. The parts that make up the 'actualities' of the phenomenon.

Being-in-the-world. How people are immersed inextricably in their everyday realities and understand themselves, other people and other things, through that immersion.

Dasein (There-Being, actualities). The 'There-Being' or 'actualities' of existence, the ontological appreciation of Being within entities.

Lived experience. The ways in which people understand themselves, other people and things, through living their life.

Ontology. The study of Being.

Ordinariness. The common bond of humanity that ties people together.

Phenomenology. A philosophical approach that continues the ontological search for the Being (Dasein, There-Being, actualities) of people and things, by exploring those things themselves.

Professorial Nursing Unit (PNU). Established and facilitated by a Professor of Nursing, a Professorial Nursing Unit is a centre providing patient care, where nursing care is the primary need and therapy.

Qualities and activities. Things that inform the aspects of the phenomenon.

2. Understanding the nature and effects of nursing

Nursing takes in a wide span of interests, because it is situated in the human world and it has people as its reason for being. Some people may become patients at some time in their lives, and some other people choose to become nurses, to care for them. Patients and nurses live out their existence in relation to one another, as humans, when they come together for purposes of caring, in nursing contexts. Nurses may be present in people's lives at birth, or death, or at times in between. Regardless of whomever else may be present, the chances are that a nurse will be there, as a helper, a healer, and a friend.

Nurses are present and active throughout people's lives, and nurses' roles, responsibilities, and ways of being are as many and varied as the situations in which they find themselves, therefore, succinct descriptions of nursing become difficult. Nurses have an interest in seeking to describe their work in relation to other people, and for this to be explicated, nurses need a method for generating these understandings. Methods are ways of finding out information about a particular area of interest, and are built on certain assumptions about the nature of knowledge and existence, and how they can be accessed in particular contexts. Nursing is about human interaction, and it can describe its own knowledge and existence, by describing the human nature of and effects of interaction between the people involved, that is nurses and patients. This assumption about the nature of nursing was the basis of the search for a suitable methodology for understanding the phenomenon of ordinariness in nursing.

After considering what the research hoped to understand in relation to the nurse-patient relationship, phenomenology was chosen as the methodology, because it was seen to contain certain underlying assumptions about the nature of human existence on which a method could be formed to explore the phenomenon of interest. More specifically, the methodology for the research was a form of hermeneutical phenomenology, in the tradition of Heidegger and Gadamer.

This chapter describes phenomenology as a methodology, by examining briefly the various types phenomenology, and by overviewing some important contributions to phenomenology by Husserl, Heidegger, and Gadamer. Even though Husserl's concept of transcendental phenomenology was not the direct basis of the method for this research, some of his ideas are included in this chapter, in acknowledgement of his original thoughts which were beginning points for the different perspectives put forward later by Heidegger and Gadamer. The chapter then establishes what the phenomena of interest to nursing are, and the connections between nursing and phenomenology are explored, before some contributions to nursing of a phenomenological nature are reviewed. Finally, a description will be given of the ways in which phenomenology informed the theoretical framework for the research, so that a methodologically congruent method could be generated.

Phenomenology: a people-valuing methodology

Although phenomenology can seek to understand any person or thing in the world, in the social sciences it is used primarily to understand people. Phenomenology was used in this research as both the methodology and the method. The catch-cry of phenomenology from its Husserlian beginnings has been: 'To the things!' (Zu den Sachen), meaning that its prime intent is to discover, explore, and describe 'uncensored phenomena' (Spiegelberg 1970 p21) of the things themselves, as they are immediately given. In this sense, I went, as the researcher, to the nurses and patients in the place in which they interacted, in order to discover, explore, and describe the participants' intersubjective understandings of their relationships and interactions.

Types of phenomenology

There is much more to phenomenology than it being simply 'the study of things', because the nature of phenomenology is multifaceted. So called 'phenomenologists' hold diverse views on epistemological and ontological questions, a realisation which caused the historian Herbert Spiegelberg (1976) to suggest that there is no school of phenomenology representing a rigid, uniform view; rather, it could be more aptly described as a 'movement.'

Spiegelberg (1970) provided a 'staggered approach' to finding common ground within the phenomenological movement, by compiling six types of phenomenology, which he explained were not mutually exclusive, but rather they were unified in a common purpose of 'giving us a fuller and deeper grasp of the phenomena' (p19).

The types of phenomenology include: 'descriptive phenomenology', which is a direct description of phenomena aimed at maximum intuitive content; 'essential (eidetic) phenomenology', which seeks to explain essences and their relationships; 'phenomenology of appearances', which attends to the ways in which phenomena appear; 'constitutive phenomenology', which studies the processes whereby phenomena become established in our consciousness; 'reductive phenomenology', which relies on suspending belief in the reality or validity of phenomena, and 'hermeneutic phenomenology', which is a special kind of phenomenological interpretation to unveil hidden meanings in phenomena.

Each type of phenomenology is related in part to the others, through complex networks of philosophical debate about key concepts. Notwithstanding the diversity of their conceptual arguments, the binding concern that all types of phenomenology share is their desire for the direct exploration of phenomena as a means of explicating Being, which is the nature of existence itself. In this research, the assumptions of an hermeneutic form of phenomenology were used, however, in acknowledgement of the original eidetic phenomenological concepts generated by Husserl, some of his work will be outlined, to show the main shifts in thought between him and Heidegger and Gadamer.

Husserl (1970 trans.) criticised Descartes for introducing into philosophy the separation between thinking substance (res cogitans) and extended substance (res extensa), thus Husserl opposed the dualism of Descartes and he sought to find a way of explaining human existence through a better method. Instead of using Cartesian doubt, which would ultimately deny the world itself, Husserl advocated a method of reduction, which would return one to phenomena of which one was conscious as legitimate concerns of philosophy. Husserl thereby extended the term 'experience' past things known by sense perception, as demanded by empirico-analytical analyses, to anything of which one was conscious. In this way, Husserl advocated a return to philosophical questions about subjectivity and consciousness, which had become offsided as concerns, because they could not be examined through the then exclusive and fashionable empirico-analytical methods of hard core science.

Husserl's commitment to the idea of transcendental phenomenology (Husserl 1980 trans.) came from his search for a science of essences, an 'apodictic beginning point, for an indubitable epistemic foundation' which in itself discovers Being (Stapleton 1983 p4). In other words, he was searching for the indisputable source of knowledge itself. Husserl used the word transcendental in the Kantian sense, to mean the conditions necessary for experience. In his view, the transcendental was neither subject or object, rather it formed the conditions that make subjective and objective experience possible. This means that he attempted to go back to find the nature of the furtherest point of things, to the point at which they could be explored as things in themselves, as the generative source of things that could later be regarded as subject or object.

The phenomenological method suggested by Husserl required that one suspend one's unquestioning acceptance of the pre-philosophical or natural attitude, which is situated in a web of relationships to things and people in the natural world, to take on the philosophical attitude, which demands to know the reasons why things are as they are. The transition from the prephilosophical to the philosophical attitude was through a phenomenological reduction, which narrowed one's attention in such a way as to be able to discover rational principles underlying the phenomenon of concern. In other words, all things already known or experienced about the phenomenon of interest were to be discounted and ignored, so that one could go to the point at which the essence of the thing itself could be made manifest.

This narrowing of focus, that is, the phenomenological reduction, otherwise known as the phenomenological epoche, was achieved by a suspension of judgement, by questioning all previous presuppositions, until further investigation was possible. Being a mathematician, Husserl gave the name 'bracketing' to this process of leaving something to one side in parenthesis. Keen to make his meaning clear for this important step in gaining phenomenological understanding, Husserl used the words phenomenological reduction, epoche and bracketing synonomously, as different metaphors explaining the same philosophical attitude.

Husserl claimed that there was a residue, which remained after bracketing; that something which remained was the ego itself. In order to escape the subject-object dualism of Cartesian thought and subsequent philosophy, Husserl referred to this ego as 'transcendental consciousness,' because it embraced both subjective and objective elements. He contended that ego could not be conceived apart from conscious life, thus consciousness was always intended towards ego. The phenomenological epoche was therefore a means by which the natural world could be reduced to a transcendental consciousness or transcendental subjectivity, through which 'consciousness was purified and only phenomena remained. Analysing the phenomena, in turn, revealed the basic structure of consciousness itself' (Husserl 1980 trans.). This meant that one needed to take everything else out of consideration, to get to the basic nature of the thing of interest.

For Husserl, every experience could be trans.formed into its essence, or eidos. Eidetic intuition meant seeing into the essence of a thing. Stapleton (1983 p40) clarified that Husserl meant eidos or essence as:

a priori, but by this he did not mean that it was supplied solely by the mind prior to empirical experience but rather that it is an ability to have an insight prior to empirical experience which is then fulfilled or 'fleshed out' by experience. In short, the eidos is the 'essential possibility' without which experience would be impossible.

Husserl defended his concept of the lived world (Lebenswelt) (1960, 1964 trans.). In response to his critics, who claimed that his theory of eidetic phenomenology was taking him away from the world of everyday experience, Husserl insisted that the lived world was the context for all experience. This context, or 'horizon,' included everything in which one experienced things, such as time, space, surrounding people, and the world itself. He reiterated that one could not be separate from the world, but that it was always there as background for all human endeavours, regardless of whether they could be judged as real or illusory.

Husserl was Heidegger's teacher and colleague, and authors (Kockelmans 1967, Spiegelberg 1970, 1976, Stapleton 1983, Sukale 1976) have elaborated on their personal and philosophical differences. Sukale (1976 p101) concluded that 'the basic difference between Husserl and Heidegger boiled down to their different interpretation of the concept of 'world.' It was as though there were different two levels; the level of the natural world, and the level below the natural world, from which all things sprang. Husserl was intent on reaching the world below, whilst Heidegger was concerned with Being-in-the-world; therefore, instead of trying to lay presuppositions to one side, Heidegger explored them as legitimate parts of Being.

Heidegger's main departures from Husserlian phenomenology were found in Heidegger's *Being and Time* (1962 trans.). Heidegger began his book with a question about Being, thus placing his search firmly in the perspective of hermeneutical enquiry. He established 'Being [as] the most universal concept' (p22) and then argued that:

the question of Being must be formulated. If it is a fundamental question, or indeed the fundamental question, it must be made transparent and in an appropriate way (p24).

Heidegger sought to establish the basis of philosophy as an historical analysis of existence, raising questions about Being and hermeneutical enquiry. Thus, Heidegger saw the task of philosophers as ontologists, seeking to unravel 'the universal structures of Being as they manifested themselves in the phenomena' (p277). Herein lies a major departure from the work of Husserl; Heidegger 'overcame the obsession with epistemology that characterises much of nineteenth and twentieth century approaches' (Hekman 1986 p 112), to pursue understanding through ontological enquiry.

In using hermeneutical enquiry to pursue the question of Being, Heidegger demonstrated effectively the nature of 'Dasein,' that is, the nature of human entities, who have some awareness of how to ask questions about Being, in as much as their Being-in-the-world as humans gives them some clues to the existence and nature of Being.

When first introduced into the text, 'Dasein' was described in this way by Heidegger (1962 trans. p27):

Thus to work out the question of Being adequately, we must make an entity—the enquirer—transparent in his own Being. The very asking of this question is an entity's mode of Being; and as such gets its essential character from what is enquired about—namely, Being. This entity which each of us is himself and which includes enquiring and the possibilities of its Being, we shall denote by the term 'Dasein.'

Heidegger began his hermeneutical enquiry into Being by examining the formal structures of questioning itself, before considering the behaviour of the questioner. In this analysis, Heidegger shifted from the question to the essential act of questioning. In so doing, Heidegger uncovered certain a priori objective and subjective forms. The final step was in arguing that to raise a question the questioner, must have some idea of what to ask. In this way, Heidegger created a hermeneutical circle that demonstrated the presupposition of the need of a knowing questioner.

Heidegger's ontological use of the hermeneutic circle, transformed the scope, meaning, and significance of it, as described previously by Scheiermacher (1977 trans.) and Dilthey (1976 trans.), by moving hermeneutics away from its sole focus on texts, to the interpretation of the human being, through the understanding of Being implicit in Dasein. Heidegger (1962 trans.) extended the hermeneutic circle to the ontological expression of Dasein, so that a fundamental ontology could be developed by an hermeneutic interplay between entities (expressions of Being) and sense (concern about Being). Essentially, this means that humans have the potential of understanding the nature of human existence, given their daily immersion in it.

For Heidegger, the hermeneutic circle aided in the interpretation of 'Dasein' itself as an understanding, caring mode of Being. 'Dasein' tied to the world the one who questioned, a place from whence no conscious separation was possible, given the nature of Being-in-the-world. In other words, it was reasoned that humans could not help but to raise questions about their existence, given their human embodiment and activities.

For Husserl, the ultimate intentional connection between the act of knowing and the thing as known, abided in 'pure consciousness,' or in transcendence of the natural attitude, whereas, for Heidegger, it was in the whole of people's precognitive awareness, by virtue of their prior understanding of Being, by being inextricably immersed within it. Schrag (in Kockelmans 1967 pp283-4) summarised it in this way:

> 'Dasein'…is a being who is intentionally related to his world in his pre-theoretical preoccupations and concerns. In all of man's practical and personal concerns a world is presupposed. To exist is to find oneself in a world to which one is related in one or several of the manifestations of care (Sorge) in one's construction and use of tools, in one's understanding and ordering of projects, or in one's encounter and dealings with other selves.

Heidegger conceptualised 'Dasein' as the kind of Being that had logos, or the potential to make manifest phenomena as they were, not so much through reason or speech, but as the power it had within itself to gather and preserve the things that were manifest in its Being. For people living their day to day lives, this gathering happened already in a fundamental, yet unobtrusive way in their everyday dealings. Hence, for Heidegger, Being was not gained through Husserl's method of eidetic reduction, rather it was already present in the concrete existence of things and people in the world, a concept Heidegger named Being-in-the-world.

Heidegger's ontological phenomenology was concerned with existence, specifically human existence, or 'Dasein', so in that sense it was existential. However, the point of departure with his approach as existential phenomenology as such, was in his emphasis on an hermeneutic, which analysed the historically situated self as a Being-in-the-world, thus it became an existential-ontological hermeneutic. For Heidegger, people were always arriving out of their past, deciding on their present, and anticipating their future, the ultimate reality of which is death; thus the seeds to understanding Being itself and its phenomena were in the historicity and temporality of people's Being-in-the-world. Put simply, this means that Heidegger believed that people's unique lives, lived through the passage of time from their births until their deaths, were the potential for understanding the nature and purposes of human existence.

Gadamer's major work, *Truth and Method* (1975), addressed the task of hermeneutics, to explore philosophically the conditions of all understanding. Attempting to find out what the human sciences really were, that is, 'what kind of insight and what kind of truth' could be found in the human sciences (p*xi*), he set up a conflict between truth and method, which needed to address the question that if human sciences went beyond method and still had truth, whether truth itself was beyond the question of method. In other words, he was interested in finding out whether a method, or way of directing understanding for finding truth, was necessary or whether truth could be accessed directly.

By exploring basic humanistic concepts, and by making an analysis of the experience of art, he sought to discover how understanding was possible. Gadamer (1975 p*xxii*) decided that all understanding is hermeneutical, because hermeneutics is the 'basic being-in motion of There-being, which constitutes its finiteness and historicity and hence includes the whole experience of the world.' This means Gadamer reasoned that questions raised in the course of daily life afforded answers that gave clues to the nature of human existence. For Gadamer, the study of hermeneutics was ontological, being ultimately connected to the study of language, wherein Being could be understood.

He resolved that the nature of the human sciences was in appreciating that all understanding is linguistic and can be thus examined through language. Like Heidegger before him, Gadamer was convinced that understanding was not an epistemological problem, but that rather it was an ontological one. This means that they both believed that understanding Being through ontology gave one the answers to questions about knowledge and truth. In avoiding Heidegger's tendency towards ontological absolutism, which claimed that Being was all there is as the source of understanding, Gadamer discussed ontology in terms of the linguisticity of all understanding and historicity. For Gadamer, Being resided in people's language and lives.

Gadamer adopted Heidegger's view of the hermeneutic circle, that it was necessary in the ontology of understanding as an 'interplay of the movement of tradition' and its consequences (Gadamer 1975 p261). He determined that the tendency of the Enlightenment to attempt to eradicate prejudice was prejudicial in itself, and that truth could be pursued by identifying the connections between truth and prejudice. He contended that it was the task of hermeneutics to make distinctions between true and false prejudices, by a process of effective historical consciousness. Gadamer suggested that effective historical consciousness was analogous to the I-Thou relationship (1975 p323), in which openness to the other and willingness to be modified, created a dialogical relationship.

Using the concept of horizon described by Husserl, as the 'range of vision that includes everything that can be seen from a particular vantage point,' Gadamer (1975 p269) determined that a 'fusing of horizons' occurs in effective historical consciousness. One's own horizon is understood in order to understand another's, and the conscious act of fusion of the two horizons is through an act of understanding, as the task of effective historical consciousness.

Gadamer (1975 trans. p350-351) used conversation as an example of the fusion of horizons, by noting that the merging of meaning that goes on is an instance of the linguisticality of understanding, as the 'concretation' of effective historical consciousness. This means that when people talk with one another, they work through their perceptions to find a place of mutual understanding. The correctness of interpretation is decided by examining the degree of 'conformity to the horizon from which the interpretation is made and the prejudices that constitute the horizon' (Hekman 1986 p115). Thus, for Gadamer and for Heidegger, understanding is ontological, having its basis in language, which is the 'House of Being.'

As the first 'phenomenologist' to expound on matters relating to phenomenology, Husserl provided a basis on which other phenomenologists could build. Using some of Husserl's concepts of horizon and lived experience, Heidegger set up the pursuit of understanding as an ontological problem, and emphasised that the world of people and things, in which people found themselves, was a legitimate part of that exploration. Gadamer continued the ontological explorations of Heidegger and conceptualised effective historical consciousness, gained through a fusion of horizons of the interpreter and the text. Although a wider view of the work of all three phenomenologists is important to the growth of the methodology itself, for the purposes of the research described in this book, the concepts of lived experience, Dasein, Being-in-the-world, and fusion of horizons, were particularly helpful in creating a method for directing enquiry.

Phenomenology as a useful method for exploring nursing

Nursing is presently seeking disciplinary status, on the basis of its unique knowledge about caring for people in their health and illness experiences. The methodological assumptions of phenomenology can be applied within nursing, as a variety of methods that will serve as a framework of enquiry to inform the discipline of nursing about phenomena of concern to it.

There is no one accepted methodology for conceptualising nursing, nor is there one method that serves its knowledge generation best or solely. A methodology has been suggested by Paterson and Zderad (1976), that of nursology, which includes intuition and rational analysis as reasoning, however, this suggestion has not been accepted uniformly by the profession. Given its relative youth in scholastic endeavours, this is not surprising for nursing. From the beginning of the 20th century the nature of nursing has been an ongoing source of documented enquiry amongst nurses. Although there is no accepted definition of nursing as such, nurses have attempted to find consensus in regard to nursing's metaparadigm.

The metaparadigm of nursing

The metaparadigm of a discipline is the fundamental ideas on which its knowledge is founded. Fawcett (1989 p5) explained that:

[t]he metaparadigm of each paradigm of each discipline...is the first level of distinction between disciplines. It is not unusual, however, to find that more than one discipline is interested in the same or similar concepts. The unique perspective of each discipline with regard to the concepts is specified by its metaparadigm.

Although there is no agreement on the nature of nursing which is reflected in an accepted definition, there is consensus on the metaparadigm of nursing. In relation to nursing's metaparadigm, Kemp (1983 p610) wrote that:

there is general agreement that the domain of nursing is person, environment, health, and nursing. By specifying the domain of nursing, research and practice should reflect common goals of providing nurses with knowledge within these four conceptual dimensions.

Nursing scholars have written about nursing using common 'domain' areas of person, health, environment, and nursing. Scholars have conceptualised nursing from their own perspectives and also from models borrowed from other disciplines. The writing is in the form of conceptual models of nursing (Hall 1964, Johnson 1980, King 1981, Levine 1973, Neuman 1982, Newman 1979, Orem 1987, Parse 1987, Paterson & Zderad 1976, Roper, Logan & Tierney 1980, Roy 1976, Travelbee 1971, Watson 1985, Wiedenbach 1964) as well as scholarly papers on a range of concerns centring on the metaparadigm areas (Abdellah et al 1960, Benner 1984, Chinn & Jacobs 1987, Fawcett 1984, Fitzpatrick & Whall 1989, Gortner 1983, Leddy & Pepper 1989, Marriner-Tomey 1989, Meleis 1985, Nightingale 1859, Parse 1987, Pearson & Vaughan 1986, Riehl & Roy 1980, Torres 1986).

Disciplines are differentiated from one another by virtue of the interest they take in various concepts and phenomena. By virtue of its scholarly discussions and writings, the discipline of nursing now has as a legacy, a pot-pourri of ideas, which can be shared and elaborated on by other nurses, be it through formal critiques or discussions. The following section overviews some phenomena of interest to nursing.

The phenomena of interest in nursing

As used in phenomenology, the word phenomena generally means any areas of interest for philosophical enquiry. Used in a way which focuses on human interests, however, phenomena can be taken to mean the subjective experiences of individuals, whatever they are and however they are interpreted by those individuals. Meleis (in Moccia 1986 p12) wrote that 'nursing phenomena are human phenomena,' including experiences and perceptions of things common to nurses and patients.

For some people, a particular phenomenon may be uncommon, extraordinary and exceedingly remarkable, whilst for others it may be common, ordinary and unremarkable. Therefore, the difference in interpretation resides with the actual people involved and their unique circumstances. For instance, the phenomenon of pain is the subjective experience of the pain and the meaning the individual attaches to it. When pain is experienced by a patient within the parameters of the nurse-patient relationship, the potential arises for the nurse to become a therapeutic agent in being with the patient to facilitate exploration of the phenomenon and to negotiate means of supporting the person throughout their experience.

Nurses are central figures in the daily dramas enacted in real life experiences of people who are dealing with their need for care. The phenomena of interest to nursing are those as identified by nurses and patients in the course of their everyday encounters, as well as more 'academic' issues considered away from clinical nursing contexts.

Phenomena identified and explored by patients and nurses in clinical contexts may be the experience of hope, grief, loss, suffering, and so on, whereas concerns generating theory outside the immediate nurse-patient relationship, may be about broader epistemological and ontological issues as they relate to nursing, such as the theory-practice nexus or the nature of nursing.

All of these phenomena are related to, and explored within, the metaparadigm of person, health, environment, and nursing. The explorations of these phenomena serve the immediate ends of relieving human suffering and enhancing patient care generally, as well as generating knowledge to bolster the disciplinary base of nursing itself.

The connections between phenomenology and nursing

It becomes apparent that there are parallels between phenomenology and nursing, when one considers that the phenomena of interest to nursing are connected intimately to the subjective experiences of patient and nurses as a people, who exist in an environment, wherein health is attained and maintained.

Phenomenological methodology has been advanced as 'an interpretive way of knowing.' Phenomenology is a type of qualitative methodology, in that it seeks to 'understand empirical matters from the perspective of those being studied' (Davis 1973 in Norris 1982 p40). Generated as a consequence of growing disillusionment with empirico-analytical ways of knowing as the only means to reflect the everyday realities of the human condition, phenomenological methodology has developed as a paradigm reflective of:

> pragmatic activity, that is, everyday understanding and practices, and the study of relational issues, [which] are distinctly different from the study of objects, as in the natural sciences...(Allen, Benner & Diekelmann 1986 p28)

Nursing and phenomenological methodology share the beliefs and values that people are whole and that they create their own particular meanings. Both:

consider all that is available in the experience under study, both subjective and objective, and strive to understand the total meaning that the experience has had for the participants. (Omery 1983 p62)

Thus it is that phenomenology and nursing are related, through their shared approaches to viewing people as subjective beings, whose objective and subjective experiences are meaningful in terms of the context in which they find themselves. Phenomenology and nursing are thus concerned with understanding the practical concerns of people as they live their day to day lives.

Understanding people in nursing through a phenomenological perspective, therefore, sheds some light on the meanings these people assign to their experiences of illness and of the nurse-patient relationship, thereby finding ways of caring that are particular to the experiencing person and in so doing adding to the theoretical base of the practice discipline of nursing.

Phenomenology is interested in people's lived intersubjective experiences in their worlds, for the ways in which they illuminate Being; therefore, both nursing and phenomenology are concerned with the interpretation of peoples' experiences in their worlds of everyday existence. Nursing viewed from a phenomenological perspective provides an illumination of the world of nurses and patients as entities, or beings of Being. The following section will describe how some nursing scholars have conceptualised nursing using phenomenological understandings.

Some phenomenological contributions by nurses

The literature to be discussed in this section will be that which acknowledges and explores explicitly a phenomenological view of the world of nursing. This is to differentiate between the writing of some nurses, who use intentionally a phenomenological perspective (Aamodt 1983, Benner 1984, Bergum 1989, Oiler 1982, 1986, Omery 1983, Parse, Coyne & Smith 1985, Paterson & Zderad 1976, Rieman 1986) and the work of other nurses, who describe a phenomenological perspective by chance or in part, by centring their work on the humanistic nature of the nurse-patient relationship (Brown 1986, McMahon & Pearson 1991, Parker 1986, Pearson 1988c, Peplau 1952, Muetzel 1988, Swaffield 1988, Travelbee 1963, 1966, 1971, Watson 1985).

Paterson (1971, 1978), Paterson and Zderad (1976), Benner (1984), and Benner and Wrubel (1989) used phenomenology as a method for generating knowledge about nursing. Paterson and Zderad used existential concepts to illustrate the existence of nurses and patients as lived experience in clinical settings, and Benner was influenced by the phenomenological perspectives of Heidegger and Gadamer to describe the knowledge embedded in expert nursing practice.

Paterson and Zderad described the lived experience of patients and nurses as a mutually rewarding process. Benner was able to show the value of practitioner knowledge to the patients as well as to the discipline of nursing. Like other phenomenological studies, Benner's work relied on the accounts of participants, who described their experiences. Missing from this important work are accounts of the nurses' partners in nursing encounters, the patients.

The rationale for, and selection of, a phenomenological method for studying nursing has been described by nurses (Aamodt 1983, Bergum 1989, Oiler 1982, 1986, Omery 1983, Parse, Coyne & Smith 1985, Rieman 1986). These nurses have been influential in heralding the joys and pitfalls of qualitative research, particularly that which uses a phenomenological approach.

Aamodt (1983) emphasised the need for inductive research to develop discovery in nursing and she also discussed the assumptions of time and space as context bound, and asked whether a study contributed to nursing. Bergum (1989) used a phenomenological method to describe the transformation from woman to mother, by asking women to talk about their lives as they became mothers. She concluded that the questions raised in the study are being lived in her own experience and that of the other women in the study, attesting to the ongoing dialogical nature of phenomenological research.

Oiler (1982, 1986) discussed phenomenology as philosophy, an approach, and method, and pointed out to nurses the subjective nature of people's realities, and the phenomenological method of bracketing, intuiting, analysing and describing as it relates to nursing. Omery (1983) used a similar approach to Oiler and compared the methodologies underlying selected quantitative and qualitative methods.

Parse, Coyne and Smith (1985) provided a detailed description of the essentials of phenomenological method and adaptations, before reporting on their study of 'The Lived Experience of Health,' which used the method described by Van Kaam (1969). Rieman

(1986) explored the meaning of a caring interaction using the existential themes of Buber and Marcel, to find existential perspectives of caring by using a method developed by Colaizzi. The net effect of these writings is in the making of meaning in people's lives and in nursing.

McPherson (1987) described her experience of being a patient, diagnosed as having diabetes. She linked her experience of being nursed to humanistic nursing, as it was described by Paterson and Zderad (1976) and centred on the intersubjective reality of the context in which she found herself. McPherson's phenomenological contribution to nursing is especially useful, given that it is from her twin realities of nurse and patient.

Gulino (1982) explored an existential approach to nursing care, as an alternative to the problem solving, which she considered to be a result of scientific progress and the concern for quantitative data. She contrasted the separation of the researcher and the object of study, as typified in problem-solving, to the mystery and involvement of reflection inherent in an existential approach to nursing care, and suggested that nursing needs to examine as many ways of knowing as is necessary, to yield insights into the complex nature of people.

Forrest (1989) used phenomenology and Colaizzi's procedure to find seven categories under two broad classifications of 'What is caring,' and 'What effects caring.' The focus of the study was the lived experience of nurses caring for patients. To do this, the researcher acknowledged intuition and subjectivity as a legitimate part of her findings on caring, in as much as phenomenology seeks to understand consciousness and subjectivity as integral to human experience.

Kretlow (1990) described a phenomenological view as one way of thinking about illness. She represented patient's views of illness as being 'alienating, creating uncertainty and feelings of despair,' (p8) and used her findings to suggest that nurses clarify their thinking about their practice and take up the role of patient advocate in the broadest sense, including advocacy of the right to hope.

Based on the notion that there is an imbalance of power in the patient-caregiver relationship, Drew (1986) studied the phenomena of exclusion and confirmation as patients' experiences. Given that the intent of the study was to uncover the experience of power imbalances, it is possible that the study's aims would have been better served by a method which used a critical perspective, for instance feminism or action research. Notwithstanding the value of the findings, this work contributes to nursing by providing an example of 'mixed methodology,' so that nurses can debate whether language such as 'reliability,' and 'subjects,' and a grounded theory method of analysis, actually constitute phenomenological research or some other form of qualitative research.

It raises the awareness that a study claiming to study phenomena is not necessarily phenomenological by virtue of being concerned with phenomena, given that the world is full of people and things given to consciousness. If a study does not rest on phenomenological understandings, and does not use a phenomenological method, it is reasonable to suggest that it may well be qualitative, but not necessarily, phenomenological.

Whereas the nursing scholars represented in this section are by no means the only nurses, who are thinking about nursing in a phenomenological way, the work of the nurses overviewed here is nonetheless influential in contributing to phenomenological research and discussion in nursing. As suggested at the outset of this section, however, there are many other nursing scholars who describe nursing from humanistic viewpoints, which are related in part to the tenets of phenomenology, in that they hold that human experience is full of intersubjective, context-laden phenomena, the nature of which needs to be uncovered in order to assist nursing in its mission to care.

According to Swanson and Chenitz (1982 p242):

> [n]o one methodological stance, in and of itself, leads to scientific discovery and theoretical breakthroughs. Therefore, in order to make any discoveries that are relevant to nursing practice, we must encourage the use of a variety of scientific approaches. Qualitative research is a systematic study of the world of everyday experience.

Nursing needs to draw on a variety of ways of knowing to reflect its uniqueness. Phenomenology is one methodology from which methods can be formed, in order to assist nursing in making available to the practice discipline of nursing that knowledge which is central to the everyday concerns of its participants.

The method used for researching ordinariness in nursing

Essentially inductive, for descriptive explorations of all phenomena including human experience, phenomenological methods attempt to investigate and describe the way things appear, whether they are perceived as free from, or as part of, human presuppositions. Phenomenology per se has no one way of finding intersubjective meaning; therefore, phenomenological research is not standardised into a single method. The unifying theme of all phenomenological research is that of attempting to return 'to the things themselves,' albeit through various paths. The following section will address the way in which phenomenology as method looks at the world to consider selected foci of interest, before describing the form of hermeneutical phenomenological method used in this research.

The literature reflects some differences in phenomenological views on the topics of 'world' and the nature of knowing and being, by presenting a variety of methods for phenomenological enquiry. No structured steps in a method are advocated by some people (Morris 1977, Psathas 1973, Schwartz & Jacobs 1979), whilst others like Patton (1980) feel that the enquiry must proceed as the experience unfolds, the only methodological consideration being that enquirers use some form of bracketing to minimise presuppositions.

Some authors claim that researchers need some framework to assist their enquiries, and thus some adaptations of 'the phenomenological method' for analysing particular phenomena by intuiting, analysing and describing (Spiegelberg 1976) have been suggested. Some of these include the Van Kaam method (1959), the Giorgi method (1975), and the Colaizzi method (1978). The methods range in specificity for guiding the researcher in a method which will uncover, supposedly, the nature of the phenomenon of interest.

A method of transformation of interpretations has been suggested by Langveld (1978). Essentially Husserlian in nature, this method raises the questions discussed already in this book about Husserl's search for essences and transcendental consciousness. The tension lies in the use of the terminology 'ground structure,' which seems to suggest certain universal principles reminiscent of positivistic understandings, an apparent contradiction for a methodology that is seated in the moment of an experience, and that concerns itself with ongoing dialogue. If one doubts that the essence of things can be found by bracketing the world, the legitimacy of this method is doubtful in describing Being within 'the things themselves.'

Thus it can be seen that there are many paths to the same end of phenomenology, that is, to the 'Beingness' of the phenomenon. A question which can be raised to any person proposing a phenomenological method is: 'How will you know what you are looking at when you are confronted with 'the thing itself?' Given that the nature of the thing is not manifest fully in the natural world, and that it requires a phenomenological method for fuller illumination, it is possible entirely that the inquirer may not recognise the thing as it appears, and, therefore, keeps searching for something that will always remain elusive.

Given the exploration of the philosophical literature, some ideas in phenomenology that informed the theoretical framework of this research were identified as 'lived experience' (Dilthey 1985 trans., Heidegger 1962, trans., Husserl 1965, 1970, 1980 trans., Gadamer 1975 trans.), 'Dasein' (Heidegger 1962 trans.), 'Being-in-the-world' (Dreyfus 1991, Heidegger 1962 trans.) and 'fusion of horizons' (Gadamer 1975 trans.). These phenomenological concepts will now be discussed in relation to their theoretical implications for the research.

Lived experience

Lived experience is awareness of life without thinking about it, a pre-reflexive consciousness of life (Dilthey 1985 trans.) that, when remembered, gathers interpretive significance. Gadamer (1975 trans.) claimed that the value of lived experience of and for people, is in its potential to join together universal and personal aspects of their worlds.

As humans living together in the daily world of the nursing unit, nurses and patients amass their experiences by virtue of living their lives. The sense nurses and patients make of their lives, and the people and things around them, is because of their lived experiences. Therefore, the concept of lived experience was integral to the theoretical framework of this research, because it informed the participants about their respective impressions of their worlds, and connected them to one another, through the commonality of their lived experiences of nursing in the nursing unit.

Dasein

Heidegger (1962 trans.) used the term 'Dasein' to denote the exploration of an entity, as a means of finding Being. Although phenomenology can search for Being in all phenomena, ontological searches in the human sciences use the human being as an entity through whom to understand Being. Heidegger felt that Being could be located and described within the questioning human. For Heidegger, the 'Dasein' of the inquirer was the beginning point of discovery of Being within an entity. 'Dasein' or 'There-Being', therefore, denotes a human means of explicating the nature of Being.

The concept of 'Dasein' informed the theoretical framework of this research, because the 'There-Being' of nurses and patients reflected some of the nature of the 'Beingness' within the phenomenon. As the researcher, I decided to use the word 'actualities,' to equate with Heidegger's concept of 'Dasein'. The reason for substituting the word 'actualities' for 'Dasein' was that I considered the word 'actualities' would have more 'user-friendly' relevance for English speaking, pragmatically oriented individuals, such as nurses, as well as for the community of people for whom the findings of this research were likely to be most helpful.

Being-in-the-world

We live out our experiences within the total context of our lives, that is, the time and space of our existence from our birth until our death. As people living within the world, we are fashioned and affected by it, so that we cannot claim to ever be free of it—nor would we want to, because our Being-in-the-world connects us to our presuppositions and the nature of Being within us.

The concept of Being-in-the-world was part of the theoretical framework of this research, because it related to the idea of lived experience and to the search for Being within our human identities as people within our worlds. Being-in-the-world, therefore, emphasised the importance of contextual features within the research and freed the participants from trying to reduce away their presuppositions, which were integral to their human nature.

Fusion of horizons

Taking into account the effects of Being-in-the-world and the ways in which we understand ourselves and other people and things, through our lived experiences and language, the Gadamerian concept of fusion of horizons attests to the understandings of Being, that take place when inquirers immerse themselves in the analysis of text, and allow the horizon of the text to fuse with the horizon of their own awareness, to form a 'fusion of horizons' (Gadamer 1975 trans.).

The concept of fusion of horizons was a part of the theoretical framework as the method through which the participants' impressions were transcribed, analysed and interpreted, to describe the nature and effects of the phenomenon of ordinariness in nursing. Essentially a method of hermeneutical phenomenology, the transcribed text of participants' accounts of their experiences in the world of the PNU, was analysed to illuminate the phenomenon of ordinariness in nursing.

The phenomenological method used in this research was one which attested to the nature of Being immersed within people's particular experiences of Being-in-the-world. Therefore, the method used made no attempts to bracket presuppositions to find essences of things, rather it acknowledged the importance of people's lived experiences by exploring the participants' worlds and the inter-subjective meanings they found within them.

The following section will describe the method in detail, by setting out its component parts in relation to one another as they emerged from the context and continued towards making the phenomenon manifest.

From context to phenomenon: manifesting the nature of the phenomenon

The search for the nature of the phenomenon of ordinariness in nursing began with the context of the people, place, and time and used their intersubjective understandings to move towards describing the phenomenon itself.

Context

The method acknowledged the importance of context, wherein and through which people made sense of their lived experiences. The method situated individuals in their particular temporo-spatial contexts, including their personal and health or illness-related circumstances.

Nurse-patient interactions

I was present as a participant observer at twenty-four nurse-patient interactions. The interactions included any nurse-patient communications that were part of the negotiated plan of care for each patient. I secured informed consent to participate from all the research participants, and the nurses involved informed me when nursing care interactions were due to happen.

Participants' impressions

All of the research participants gave their impressions of the nurse-patient interactions and related areas of interest. After each interaction, I recorded my impressions in my journal, including pre-interview and post-interview notes, some demographical information, and a full account of the interaction. I interacted with each nurse and patient as appropriate to each interaction and noted the extent and nature of my interactions in my journal as part of my impressions.

After each interaction, I audiotaped a conversation with each patient, in which the only structuring guides were:

> 'I was with you when you interacted with (the nurse) this morning. What did you like about being with (the nurse) this morning? What didn't you like about being with (the nurse) this morning?
> It seems likely that what happened was a fairly usual occurrence for (the nurse). Is there anything about being with (the nurse) that was special for you?'

When audiotaping a conversation with each nurse after the respective nurse-patient interactions, the only structuring guide was:

> 'I was with you when you were with (the patient) this morning. Tell me your impressions of being with (the patient) this morning.'

The audiotapes were transcribed and, with my journal notes, became text for an hermeneutical interpretation of the respective nurse-patient interactions.

Qualities and activities

The text was analysed to find the main aspects illuminating the phenomenon. Initially, this was done by using a computerised qualitative data analysis package, to search for frequently recurring words and phrases. Following the initial search, I read and re-read the data to immerse myself fully in the contextual features of each interaction. A large set of qualities and activities emerged from the initial searches of the impressions, which were then grouped into aspects.

Aspects

After further reading of the text, I merged my own impressions with those arising from the text, to create a 'fusion of horizons,' to interpret the meaning of the phenomenon. Eight main aspects emerged from this process, which will be explained in detail later in this book.

Actualities of the phenomenon of ordinariness in nursing

Having arrived at the aspects of the phenomenon, I acknowledged the need to go beyond the external qualities and activities of the entities of the phenomenon, to seek the nature of the thing itself— which is the ultimate intent of any phenomenological method. To try to explain the nature of the aspects themselves was tantamount to Husserl's search for words to articulate 'essence' and of Heidegger's search to articulate 'Dasein.' After further immersion in the text, I used it and my own experiences of Being-in-the-world to adopt the concept of 'fusion of horizons' (Gadamer 1975 trans.), to come to insights whereby I was able to find words to portray some 'actualities' of the nature of Being, as it was embodied within the nurses and patients in the research. The actualities that emerged from this process of 'effective historical consciousness' will be explained in detail later in this book.

The process of finding meaning in each interaction

The theoretical framework underlying the processes for under- standing the participants' impressions gained from the research context, guided the way in which I made sense of using the phenomenological method. The method reflected the assumptions of a phenomenological methodology which values the concepts of lived experience, Dasein, Being-in-the-world and fusion of horizons.

The process of finding meaning in each interaction was that, as set out previously in the description, of the process from the context to the generation of the qualities and activities. The process involved analysing the text to find qualities and activities within each nurse- patient interaction

The interpretation of the meaning of each interaction was shared and checked at the time of conversation with the patients and nurses. A draft of each set of interactions was given to respective nurses for them to check the validity of my impressions against their own impressions of the interactions and to offer feedback on their perceptions. Thus, the participants validated their own impressions of their lived experiences throughout the meaning-making phase of the research process.

The process of finding meaning across interactions

The process for finding meaning across interactions was as described previously, from the context through to the description of actualities of the phenomenon. The process began with revisiting the qualities and activities that emerged from the initial meaning-making processes and ended with an articulation of some effects of the phenomenon of ordinariness in nursing.

After further re-immersion in the text, I gained insights from the fusion of my horizon with that of the text, and I grouped the qualities and activities into aspects of the phenomenon, expressed in the words: facilitation; fair play; familiarity; family; favouring; feelings; fun and friendship.

At this stage, it was acknowledged that the nature of the phenomenon was still not explicated as the 'Beingness' of ordinariness in nursing. All phenomenological methods assert an intention to go 'to the thing itself,' by seeking the nature of Being (ontological) within the entity (ontic), so a further re-immersion in the text with the insights already gained, created a new fusion of horizons, which emerged as '-ness' words that portrayed the 'innerness' of each of the aspects, these being: 'allowingness', 'straightforwardness', 'self-likeness', 'homeliness', 'favourableness', 'intuneness', 'lightheartedness' and 'connectedness'.

Having arrived at the actualities of the phenomenon, the nature of the phenomenon had been explicated, as far as the participants' impressions could be interpreted, and my abilities to use a phenomenological method allowed. The effects of the phenomenon were then to be explicated.

From phenomenon to context: manifesting the effects of the phenomenon

In considering the effects of the phenomenon, I returned to a methodological assumption of phenomenology that asserts that, in order to know the nature of the thing of interest, one goes to the thing itself. If one goes to the phenomenon and searches out its nature, and if one can assume that one has illuminated the thing intended, the effects of its nature can only be the effects of the thing itself; it cannot be anything else other than itself. This line of reasoning is in line with Heidegger (1962 trans.), who was unable to explicate Being through a temporal analysis; however, he referred to Being as 'Es' (Itself). Therefore, if Being is itself, in moving from the context to find the nature of the phenomenon it was necessary to move from the phenomenon back towards the context, to locate the effects.

Being is within context and context is within Being; they are one in the same and cannot be something different from one another; therefore, the nature of the phenomenon reflected its effects. I conceptualised as a mirror image, the move from context to phenomenon to find the nature of the thing, and the move from the phenomenon to context to find the effects of the thing. The nature of the phenomenon within the actualities of the phenomenon reflected back towards the qualities and activities as effects that emerged out of the context. Thus, the effects of the phenomenon of ordinariness in nursing were those very qualities and activities which comprised the aspects of the phenomenon. The effects of the phenomenon of ordinariness in nursing were the respective qualities and activities of each aspect, which will be described later in this book.

From the time of Husserl, phenomenology has developed many divisions and philosophical debates within itself, which have differed in the most part, on the methods by which Being could be explicated. Nurses have used phenomenological perspectives, most often those requiring some form of bracketing as proposed by Husserl, however, other forms of phenomenology are becoming apparent in the work of other scholars such as Paterson and Zderad (1976), Benner (1984), and Benner and Wrubel (1989).

This chapter described the research methodology of phenomenology and its relation to the phenomenon of interest. In considering phenomenology as methodology, this chapter examined the nature of phenomenological methodology evident in the works of Husserl, Heidegger, and Gadamer, some existing phenomenological research in nursing, and the ways in which a form of hermeneutic phenomenology informed the theoretical framework for this research into the phenomenon of ordinariness in nursing.

The method emphasised the importance of context in finding meaning in the phenomenon of ordinariness. Beginning with the context and the participants' impressions of the nurse-patient interactions, qualities and activities were recognised as ways of finding meaning within each interaction. The process for finding meaning across each interaction required sequential re-immersion in the text and in the horizon of the researcher's own experiences, to find eight main aspects across all interactions, from which eight actualities were described as the nature of the phenomenon itself.

In order to find the effects of the phenomenon of ordinariness in nursing, the nature of the phenomenon was revisited and as the phenomenon can only be a reflection of its own Being, the effects of ordinariness in nursing were recognised as being the very qualities and activities that comprised the aspects of the nature of the phenomenon itself.

Phenomenology, as a people-valuing methodology, has been used by nurses as a set of underlying assumptions on which to discover, explore and describe phenomena of interest to nursing. This chapter described phenomenology as one way of understanding nursing, by suggesting that it was a methodology with the potential for connecting a research context to a method, which could emphasise the importance of what Being-in-the-world of the nursing setting meant to each of the research participants. In accordance with such a methodology, the phenomenological method used in the research to be described in this book was a means of discovering the nature and effects of the phenomenon as it was illuminated by an hermeneutical interpretation of the text, which was in turn derived from the participants' actual lived experiences.

PART 2

Stories

3. Andrew's nurse-patient interactions

Introducing Andrew

Andrew began his nursing career in 1985. Prior to studying nursing, he gained a Bachelor of Agricultural Science, travelled overseas for a year, and had a managerial job with Kentucky Fried Chicken. When he first applied for nursing, he didn't really know if his heart was in it; but the more he thought about it and worked in it, the more it seemed right for him.

Andrew thinks that 'nursing is about helping people at all different levels: physically, emotionally, whatever. It is about being with people, talking with people and just helping basically, trying to get them to get back to the goals they desire and helping them to get what they want out of life.' In his future, Andrew would 'love to be where there is a bit of a challenge.' He wants to be somewhere where he can contribute to the profession and do something that helps to show the value of nursing.

Introducing Donald

Donald was born on 3 March 1926. He lives with his wife in a comfortable unit and they have a supportive family network. Donald has been in and out of the Professorial Nursing Unit (PNU) for eight months or so, to assist him with his diabetes and chronic obstructive airways disease. Recently, he has had the toes on his left foot removed to treat an ulcerating, necrotic (dead tissue) area and he is now ambulant.

Andrew and Donald: a story about an aseptic dressing

I notice the screens around Donald and I can tell by the talking that his dressing is being done. I peep in through Donald's curtains at the end of his bed. Donald is grimacing with pain. His wife, Betty, is standing beside him, holding his hand and speaking softly to him. Andrew and Veronica (the nurse assisting) are taking the dressing down carefully and encouraging Donald to see it through. I walk in through a partition in the curtain to the top of Donald's bed and slip quietly in on the empty side opposite Betty. I don't comment. I crouch down at Donald's head level and stand in close looking at his left foot.

Andrew is removing the dressing carefully to reveal a large, open area at the end of Donald's foot, where his toes used to be. The amputated area is open and bright pink. Greyish spots indicate where his toes were connected. The remainder of his foot is pink with large areas of purplish skin, which indicate ischaemia (a low blood supply). All in all, to the uninitiated, it could be conceived as a fairly horrendous sight.

I am aware of the acceptance of the sight of Donald's foot by all the people there. Betty is saying that she thinks it looks better than yesterday. Donald wants his glasses to look for himself. I get them off his table and buff them on my dress and hand them to him. He puts them on and leans forward in interest. His leg is shaking all the time. He has been commenting on the stinging from the solution, but as he sits forward his interest in his foot seems to calm him. He doesn't comment on the appearance of his foot.

I wonder to myself: 'How would his own foot look to him. How must it feel to lose a part of yourself and to continue on without it in pain?' Behind this screen, there is unanimous acceptance of the sight and encouragement for Donald's endurance throughout the procedure.

Donald has had Morphia intramuscularly in preparation for the dressing procedure, but the stinging seems so awful. He is sucking in air and whistling it out and it reminds me of the pain I felt in labour. Even though we are all here for him, it is still his own private agony. Donald's pain, the sight of the wound, the loving tenderness of his wife, the careful dressing by Andrew, the silent vigil by Veronica, all of it seems remarkable to me. Behind the screens we are together in a potentially horrific encounter helping Donald through his pain, assisting him by being there with encouragement, company, and skill. I stop in my head for a moment and take it in.

The dressing is over and Andrew places soaked sterile pads gently on the top of Donald's foot, telling him they are there to keep the foot moist until the doctor attends. Donald comments on the doctor's attendance, saying: 'He'd better not be late!'

Andrew looks up and comments that Donald had two beautiful women to look after him. Betty says: 'Don't you think I'm beautiful

Andrew?!' 'Oh yes,' he says, indicating towards Betty and myself. 'Doesn't Veronica get a mention?' I ask. 'No, I'm just here', she jokes, and so the repartee continues for a minute or so taking the attention right off all the intensity and industry going on at the left foot end of Donald's being.

Andrew continues to place dry pads over Donald's foot and to tape them loosely there. As I am leaving, Andrew and Veronica are talking about the requirements for the dressing after the doctor has been, Betty is receiving a kiss on the cheek from Donald, and they are smiling at one another. Andrew comments on how well Donald tolerated the procedure. We all agree.

Interpretations

Using the method I have explained previously in Chapter 2 I found that eight main qualities and activities emerged, when I analysed the text relating to the interaction between Andrew and Donald, which appeared to illuminate the phenomenon of ordinariness in nursing. The qualities and activities were those things that the nurses and patients were doing, and how they were doing them, and in the case of the interaction between Andrew and Donald they were: acknowledging the relevance of family affiliations; expressing 'family-like' ties; expressing affection and liking; enjoying a sense of humour; appreciating skilful nursing care; tolerating one another's humanness; relating to one another's humanness; and acknowledging the polarity of human feelings. Each of these qualities and activities will be discussed, because they were interpreted to be of importance in the context.

Acknowledging the relevance of family affiliations. This was expressed often by Donald in respect to the closeness he treasured with his wife. He appreciated the help Andrew gave him, but he differentiated between what Andrew was able to do for him, and the help his wife had been to him throughout his painful experiences. For Donald, his wife was the person from whom he received most assistance.

> *'Well, he [Andrew] made me feel good, but nowhere near as good as my wife could make me feel. If it wasn't for my wife I would never have got through it.'*

However, Donald acknowledged his appreciation of Andrew's care, especially of Andrew's thoughtfulness, when Donald and Betty reconsecrated their marriage vows in a ceremony in the PNU Donald recounted emotionally:

'He put a notice on the door "Do Not Disturb!". It was very thoughtful.'

Expressing 'family-like' ties. Even though, in Donald's estimation, Andrew could not compare with Betty in terms of ultimate help throughout his hospitalisation, Andrew received the highest accolade from Donald, who said:

> *'Yeah, yeah. Andrew and I get on really well together. I'd say he was more or less like a brother.'*

Expressing affection and liking. Donald was keen to give each person who interacted regularly with him a score out of ten, to reflect his appreciation of their care. Of Andrew he said:

> *'I'd give him ten out of ten'*

A high score was assigned to nurses with whom Donald interacted most frequently, because he felt he had become most familiar with them. Donald said:

> *'They had more to do with me than the others, really, when they did the dressings and that...I'd give Janice ten out of ten and the others eight out ten...I just gave them eight out of ten because I don't think they were quite as good as Andrew and Janice and Elizabeth. They [Andrew, Janice, and Elizabeth] had more to do with me than the others.'*

The nurses were not the only people Donald scored in appreciation. In relation to the person who came around daily to help with the menus he said:

> *'She was very nice. I've got to give her some points. She'd get ten out of ten, too, because she was very jovial. She got on well with my wife, too.'*

Acknowledging the relevance of family affiliations extended to Andrew as well. Andrew realised how important Donald's wife was to Donald's recovery and he included Betty in Donald's world in the PNU. In relation to the effect of Betty's presence during the painful dressing procedure, Andrew said:

> '...also knowing though that when his wife's there it does help a lot with Donald with his pain...His wife being there helped. Even Donald himself knew it had to be done...Donald understood and Betty understood, like everyone knew, that it was just a matter of waiting for it to heal.'

Enjoying a sense of humour. Donald enjoyed a sense of fun in the people who cared for him. The enjoyment of joviality was expressed by Donald, who said of Andrew:

> *'He was always very jovial. We used to give one another a lot of cheek about football. Andrew was [an] Essendon [supporter], I was [a]*

Collingwood [supporter], and we used to throw a lot of rubbish at one another. Yeah, we'd have a great discussion about it.'

Appreciating skilful nursing care. Notwithstanding all the human qualities Donald appreciated in nurses, he was also aware of competent nursing work. Donald said:

> *'Well, he [Andrew] was always very conscientious in his work. He did his job very well, and also Elizabeth, when I first went in the first time, but Andrew is probably the main one...He is always very conscientious in his job and we get along very well together...Very good, yeah. I was always very confident when Andrew was doing the job. I knew that it would be done properly...He is very gentle in handling it, not to hurt the wound. He could have been a lot rougher with it.'*

Donald also made special mention of Janice.

> *'Yeah. I'd have to give praise to Janice, when she took the dressing off that foot after the operation. It was a mean job...There was a lot of pain. They [Janice and a helper] got it off in the finish. It was a big job to get it off, about two and a half hours...Very gently. A little bit at a time.'*

Tolerating one another's humanness. Donald remarked on the less than perfect ways he noticed sometimes in the nurses. He accepted their fallibility, because he acknowledged and tolerated their humanness. Donald said of one of the nurses:

> *'Her [the nurse's] personality was very good the first time I was in, but the second time she was getting tired before she went on holidays. She was getting forgetful. She'd go away to get something and go away and forget all about it. When she'd return she'd say, just, 'I'd forgot'. She was getting a bit tired before she went on her holidays, but she was very conscientious.'*

and

> *'They were all very good; got a bit slack sometimes, but still they got there. They're busy too and they can't treat one patient all the time. They've got a lot of patients to think of as well as me.'*

Relating to one another's humanness. Andrew related strongly with the pain Donald was enduring. He had come to know Donald well and it was not easy for Andrew to tend to Donald's dressing, knowing that he was causing him pain, and wondering whether the wound would heal successfully. Andrew commented:

> 'I think I felt sorry for Donald, because he'd been through so much and he'd been in for so long, and the saga, as you know, had gone on for a long time about trying to save the foot, lose the foot, save the foot. And seeing the large skin flap hanging down and realising how painful it would have been for him. Knowing that Donald's

not a guy that, well he doesn't show his pain. Donald would break his leg and still wouldn't complain. So realising, for Donald, to show that he was in pain, then it must be hurting a hell of a lot. This particular day we'd sort of given him everything we could. I knew that it had to be done...I mean it's not nice hurting someone, well not hurting someone, but to be causing discomfort to someone that you know so well. But, knowing for a good outcome, you have to do it. You know what I mean. It wasn't being done for no reason...The end result was worth it. If you saw the end result, it's beautiful.'

Acknowledging the polarity of human feelings. Andrew was willing to acknowledge that the sight of Donald's wound was horrifying initially for him and that he questioned the value of the operation and the pain to which Donald was being subjected over the prolonged healing period. Andrew acknowledged his feelings of ambivalence and relief at the final outcome, when he said:

'Oh I was pretty horrified when I saw it. Yeah, I was pretty horrified. I remember thinking 'Oh my God, this is never going to heal!' We all thought that he was going to be here for months and months and this might never heal. But, the first couple of times, I was wondering if it was worth it, the pain we were causing Donald, and the trauma. I was thinking "Is it worth doing? Would it be better to maybe just chop the whole leg off?" But, I mean it was Donald's decision to go through that operation. Donald wanted to keep his heel, so as it turned out it worked good.'

Andrew expressed his surprise to Donald that the wound healed so fast, but he did not share his feelings of initial horror with him. Rather, he talked with colleagues about how he felt, and used them as 'sounding boards.' Andrew said:

'I'm pretty sure I told him I was surprised it healed so fast. I don't think I would have told him [of the feelings of horror]. Yeah, I use them [my colleagues] as sounding boards. Peter, Janice and I bounce off each other quite a lot. At the time Janice and myself were working together, and Janice and I used to bounce off each other quite a lot. Peter also, because Peter's done a lot of wound healing and you sort of bounce off each other, because you have to verbalise it. I mean you keep it [inside yourself] to a certain extent inside, but I find myself, it's good for me to be able to say it. I mean, people say 'How can you say that?' I mean, I'm not putting people in boxes. I just say something and then its gone.'

Conclusions

There was acceptance of the sight of Donald's foot by all the people present at the dressing. The people present had a right and reason to be there, either through family attachment, or as professional carers. Donald felt close to his wife first and foremost, but he also felt an affinity with the nurses. Even though Donald was aware of us, the dressing change was his own private agony. Behind the screens, we were together in a potentially horrific encounter, assisting him by easing his pain and by being there with encouragement, company and skill. At the closure of the procedure, Andrew's use of humour and lightness was refreshing. It was like a rest from the anguish everyone present had sensed, to some extent. The humour was well placed and tactfully done, so that it created a diversionary relief for us all.

His wife and his home were most important for Donald. In relation to the nursing staff, Donald decided who he liked by judging their degree of joviality, the way in which they acknowledged and valued his wife, and their competence as nurses. It seemed as though he connected his liking of people to the way in which they manifested these favoured qualities. The person who recorded Donald's daily meal preferences was always welcomed by him, regardless of how he was feeling, because she was able to make him feel good with her joviality. Andrew was liked by Donald because of his skill and knowledge, but the most outstanding things that caused Donald to call him 'brother' were his friendly attributes of fun and cheek, which they both enjoyed together. Donald equated most strongly with the nurses he knew best. He understood when some of them became forgetful and tired, knowing that they were busy or that they were due for a holiday. He allowed them to be less than perfect, because he knew them as people.

Andrew had come to know Donald over several admissions to the unit; therefore, he was able to judge that Donald must have been in agony, when he showed that he was having any pain at all. Andrew felt sorry for the pain Donald was experiencing, and for the part he was playing in causing it. He was as merciful as possible to Donald, by giving him analgesics and emotional support, while he tended the dressing gently and skilfully; but Andrew still felt fearful that the wound would take a long to heal, if at all. Andrew questioned with his colleagues the value of the treatment being given to Donald's foot, and he used them as sounding boards to express his horror and fears. Andrew did not tell Donald that the sight of the wound after surgery was horrifying to him, but he hinted to him that it may take a long time to heal. Andrew respected the love Donald and Betty had for each other and the effect Betty had in calming Donald and he demonstrated this by including Betty in the dressing procedure and providing them both with privacy.

It was the things they did together that made the relationship between Donald and Andrew special. For instance, Donald enjoyed the familiarity of the things he and Andrew shared: 'We used to give one another a lot of cheek' 'We used to throw a lot of rubbish at one another' 'We'd have a great discussion about it.' There was a two way relationship built an commonalities such as mutual respect and joviality. They gave and took from each other, things like jokes and discussions about the wound care, and their respective families. But, underlying it all, was the necessity to dress a painful wound, to wait for healing, to keep Donald's general health stable, and to live day to day and week to week, together in the nursing unit. They saw each other's humanity, and they accepted and respected it. Donald and Andrew kept going forward together, because that was what it was all about, getting better and going home again.

Introducing Jim

Jim was born on 13 June 1920. He lives with his wife and they have three children. Jim was admitted to the PNU to recover from a transurethral retrograde prostactectomy. He had a bladder washout recently for retained blood clots. Jim was taking oral hypoglycaemic agents, but he was experiencing persistently high blood sugars and loss of weight from self-enforced dietary restrictions. He is presently being stabilised on insulin and learning to self-administer insulin and to monitor his own blood sugar levels.

Andrew and Jim: a story about helping to learn

It is a sunny morning. There is a sense of lightness in the unit. When I locate Andrew, he is sitting on the bed next to Jim. Another nurse is sitting on the other side of Jim. She is watching how Andrew teaches Jim about giving his insulin. I sit down quietly on a chair opposite them and Andrew keeps talking to Jim.

Jim is a thin man with glasses. Today he is wearing a blue check shirt and black trousers. His eyes are wide and he is attentive fully to what Andrew is saying. Andrew speaks at a normal conversational pace and pitch, and holds an insulin syringe in front of Jim as he demonstrates the markings. Andrew describes and demonstrates systematically the procedure and then tells Jim that it is his turn to handle the syringe and insulin vial.

Jim picks up the syringe and Andrew prompts him with questions such as: 'What are you going to do first?' 'What do you do next?'

'Where are the injection sites?' Andrew does not rush Jim; he gives ample time for Jim to think, reply and act. Andrew affirms Jim's correct responses and clarifies other aspects, such as the width of tissue on the arm and thigh, in which the injections can be placed.

Jim asks questions such as: 'Do I put it on the outside of the leg?' 'If I'm having twenty units, can I have ten in the morning and ten at night?' Andrew listens and replies, being careful not to introduce too much information at one time. He says several times that it is important not confuse Jim with too much information and suggests that Jim only read the first few pages of the instructional booklet at this stage, because it is information they have dealt with already and extra information could be 'a bit too much' right now.

The lesson goes smoothly. Jim and Andrew are talking together and checking one another's perceptions throughout the interaction. At the end of the lesson, Andrew tells Jim that he has done well, especially with three people watching him. 'Yes' he replies proudly, 'I didn't even shake!' Andrew continues to confirm some points and makes the comment: 'There you are, I'm shaking now,' and we all grin together. Andrew suggests that Jim might like to show his wife how to manage the procedure, when she visits this afternoon. Andrew assures Jim that he'll be there if he needs him. 'You can impress her with your knowledge,' says Andrew. 'That would be a good idea,' beams Jim.

Interpretations

Andrew was helping Jim to manage to give himself his own insulin injections. Andrew realised that Jim had misunderstood previous information given to him by health professionals, because Jim had restricted his food intake and lost a great deal of weight, not realising that he had become insulin dependent. Not realising that no amount of dieting would relieve his hyperglycaemia, Jim had obeyed dutifully his doctor's instructions to restrict carbohydrate. Jim was a man who was willing to do as he was told, with minimal rationale. Andrew was teaching Jim about injecting his own insulin and about his diabetes generally.

Three main themes emerged from an analysis of the text relating to the interaction between Andrew and Jim, which were: helping to learn; valuing the importance of home; and approving commendable human qualities

Helping to learn. The main reason for the interaction between Andrew and Jim, was to teach Jim how to inject his own insulin, therefore, the main theme was that of Andrew helping Jim to learn. The success of the teaching was borne out by Jim's comments.

> *'Andrew is quite a good demonstrator and he's willing to help at anything. So I'm quite pleased with him. Everything seems to go alright. I understood everything he told me to do. Everything seemed to be alright, no worries about him at all…So far I can remember what to do. As long as it keeps in there [indicating his head] that's the main thing. I think I'll be right. Well, it's easier for somebody to show me what to do than reading. You might read something, but it doesn't stick in your head as somebody showing you. It helped me a lot with Andrew showing me what to do. I think he did a good job.'*

Andrew was pleased that Jim was feeling confident enough to teach his new found knowledge and skills to someone else. He was willing to share his role of teacher with Jim. Andrew said:

> *'He's pretty confident, because he's going to teach his wife now, so that's good.'*

Valuing the importance of home. Jim knew that the real test of his new found knowledge and skill, would be when he went home to his usual lifestyle, and it was important for him to feel that he could make the transition successfully from the unit to his home.

> *'Well, I've been on a diet here. It hasn't really changed my life. I haven't noticed it yet. I suppose when I do get home under my own power and that sort of thing, well, there will be a certain amount of change. I love going for holidays and that sort of thing. With a tablet, you just pop a tablet in your mouth and that's it. But with insulin, you've got to watch what you're doing a bit more and keep it at the right temperature…It's just getting into that routine again.'*

Approving commendable human qualities. Jim appreciated Andrew's teaching skills, but there was more about Andrew that he valued, which he was not able to articulate clearly.

> *'He sort of told me every step of the procedure, you know, it makes it easier. He has some way about him, that for me it seemed to stick in your head more. He's got a way about him. He makes you feel more at ease.'* [Jim became tearful at this point.]

Andrew appreciated the human qualities about Jim, which helped him to facilitate his work as nurse. He said:

> 'He's good. He's very accepting. He had a bladder washout yesterday; he got obstructed with a few clots, so I think he felt confident with me, because I was the one that was doing it [the bladder washout] with him. That tends to build up a bit of confidence. Even with the bladder washout yesterday, he seemed to be accepting, very easy going. I mean, you could tell he was

getting a bit sacred, when he started to feel his bladder and it was causing a bit of discomfort, you could tell, but he said "Oh no, I think it's alright."...It [the lesson] went well I think. Jim seemed to pick it up pretty well and he was interested. He's a pretty easy man to talk to. He's pretty accepting.'

Conclusions

Jim was a man who trusted the words and deeds of professionals, that is why he had lost so much weight trying to get his blood sugar levels down. He was told to give up certain foods, which he did dutifully and without explanation, and he could not understand why his blood sugars were still high. Jim faced the prospect of introducing the self-administration of insulin and blood glucose monitoring into his lifestyle. He was willing to try this and was pleased with Andrew, whose teaching he appreciated. When Andrew was teaching him, Jim was totally absorbed in the learning.

The lesson went smoothly. Jim and Andrew talked together and checked one another's perceptions throughout the interaction. At the end of the lesson, Andrew told Jim he had done well, especially with three people watching him. Jim replied proudly that he didn't even shake. Andrew continued to confirm some points and made the comment that he had begun to shake himself. Andrew was willing to acknowledge his own nervousness. It was OK for him to show that he was human too, and that shaking was a natural response to the situation.

Andrew liked Jim; he enjoyed teaching him. It was important to Jim that his wife was included and that he demonstrated to her that he was coping with the new information and practice. Andrew understood this and encouraged him by saying that he was ready to teach his wife. It mattered to Jim that he understood and could manage, because he wanted to continue doing with his wife the things he enjoyed. Andrew acknowledged Jim's wife's part in his education and included her by suggesting Jim was ready to teach her about insulin administration. This not only included her, but it tipped the 'power balance' in Jim's favour, so that Jim felt he had some knowledge of, and control over, his own body.

It was the beginning of his tuition and Jim had much to learn; Andrew knew this and introduced information at the rate he thought Jim could manage. Andrew understood that even though Jim had much to learn, he had always striven to follow the advice he had been given. He acknowledged Jim's receptivity to treatment and learning. It was not that Andrew wanted Jim to be an unquestioning patient, but that he appreciated Jim's attentiveness to what he had to say, and his willingness to put it into action. Andrew seemed to be able to gain Jim's confidence and Andrew assumed that it had to do with his success in unblocking Jim's catheter previously. Jim was appreciative of the way in which Andrew instructed him, but he was unable to explain just what it was that made him say of Andrew: 'He's got a way about him. He makes you feel at ease.'

Introducing Josephine

Josephine was born on 15 August 1911. She lives alone in a comfortable unit, within walking distance of the city. Josephine was admitted to hospital after a left brainstem cerebrovascular accident. Previously, she has had bilateral hip replacements. She is in the PNU to improve her walking prior to her discharge from the hospital.

Andrew and Josephine: a story about wanting to go home

Andrew and I enter the four bed room. Visitors are gathering. It is about 11.40 am. There are four people around a woman, who is sitting up in the first bed; two of the younger people are browsing through her magazines. We go to Josephine's bed and Andrew begins to screen the bed, telling her that he has come to look at her ankle dressing.

Josephine is a thin, straight woman. She has an expressionless face. This morning she has been to the physiotherapy and occupational therapy departments and she has not long arrived back in her room. Andrew helps her to lie on the bed by assisting her legs as she swings her body around. He pulls the remaining screen and prepares the dressing trolley.

He says that he hears she may be concerned about the ulcer and she says she is not worried particularly. He takes the first piece of Duoderm (a sterile wound application) down and tells her that the wound is 'looking fine; it is about the size of a one cent piece.' He asks her whether she would like to look at it and she declines. She says the district nurse has been happy with its progress.

Andrew realises that he needs a pair of scissors and excuses himself to go to get them. Seconds later, the screens open and a young woman walks in. She greets Josephine and then she introduces herself to me. 'I am Alicia,' she says to me. 'I am Bev,' I reply. She asks Josephine how she is feeling, and when Andrew returns, she comments to him that the ulcer looks good. They talk about another patient in the ward and Josephine lies quietly. Alicia tells Josephine she will go now and as she leaves Josephine says: 'Thank you doctor'.

The sun is streaming through the window and bathing the bed in warm light. I comment that it feels good on my back. Josephine nods. For the most part, Josephine lies quietly with one hand against her face. Andrew continues to dress the ulcer and he tells her that he will replace the Duoderm, so that it can stay in place for about six days or so. She says she thinks she may not be in the PNU then, so I say that it might be the district nurse, who looks at it next. She says she is not really sure when she is due to go home, but she thinks it might be soon.

Andrew asks her whether she remembers how the ulcer started. She can't remember bumping it. Andrew says he will look at the other ankle to see how it is going. She says it should be almost healed now, because it was small before. He takes off the dressing and confirms her suspicion. 'It is miniscule,' he says, 'But I'll replace the Duoderm, because the skin looks fragile.' She nods. At some point in the interaction, Josephine becomes more 'with us' and when Andrew talks she smiles. It is a noticeable difference from her fairly quiet and inanimate attitude thus far.

The second dressing is in place and she comments on going home. Andrew tells her that she is making good progress generally, but that she is tilting a little bit to the left when she walks, so she will need to practice that to be ready for home. He asks her whether she wants to sit out of bed and she says she will. He moves the wheelchair and she asks for her walking stick. She needs to go to the toilet before lunch, so he walks beside her, at her pace, up the corridor to the toilet. They continue to chat as they walk.

Interpretations

Josephine was recovering from a stroke and she had been admitted to the PNU for final rehabilitation, before going home. She was very keen to go home and appeared to be resentful of having to be in the unit. In this interaction, Andrew attended to Josephine's ulcer dressings on her ankle and talked with her generally about how she felt she was coping.

The method of analysis revealed five main qualities and activities in the text relating to the interaction between Andrew and Josephine. The qualities and activities were appreciating skilful nursing care;

approving commendable human qualities; valuing the importance of home; relating to the other's situation; and acknowledging the importance of company and talking.

Appreciating skilful nursing care. Josephine appreciated the skill with which Andrew tended the dressing of her ankle ulcers. She said:

> *'Well, he was very...He did a good dressing on my leg. It was very soothing and I think he did a very good job. I don't know really, whether it was any different really. But he is very, very, careful. I couldn't feel anything while he was doing it really.'*

Approving commendable human qualities. Josephine acknowledged that she liked the qualities of the nurses in the unit, when she said:

> *'They are all very kind. Very nice.'*

Valuing the importance of home. Home was important to Josephine; it was so important for her, that she assumed that everyone would agree with her. She said:

> *'Oh yes, well naturally, everyone likes being in their own home.'*

Andrew valued Josephine's need to go home. He found it totally reasonable that Josephine would be feeling somewhat negative about her transfer to the nursing unit, if she thought she was well enough to go home directly. Andrew explained:

> 'I think the main concern with her is that she really wants to go home. Yes, I really don't think that she's accepted being in hospital at this present stage, which is pretty true, because she really is well enough, but she is still a bit unsafe walking. And, you know, I don't know if she has accepted that fact...I think she is really missing home...It was the first time I'd actually met Josephine. Yesterday she was very unhappy about coming here, because she thought she was well enough to go home, so there was quite a negativity about being in the unit. But, I mean, that's OK. There's nothing wrong with that. She does not have to like being in the unit and it's understandable that she might be feeling some negativity.'

Relating to the other's situation. Not only was Andrew understanding of Josephine's initial negativity about being in the unit and wanting to go home, he was also able to relate to her need to be given a chance to accept her present circumstances. Andrew suggested:

> 'Just give her space. I mean, everyone needs their space. If you are ranting into them "Oh, you've got to be here for this, this, this and

this!" it's no good. You've got to give them space and give them a chance to accept it or, you know, they might never accept it fully, but just give them a chance to think about it and back off a bit. The harder you push them in that circumstance, the further you are likely to push them away from you.'

Acknowledging the importance of company and talking. It was the first time Andrew had interacted with Josephine and he felt it was important to get to know her by talking with her. Andrew said:

'I think I did talk a lot more [talking] at the start, because I was told that she was worried about it [the ulcers]. I thought I had to reassure her that it looked really good. I probably did talk more than usual during a dressing, because I wanted to show her that it was going fine. But you can definitely sense it, that she is not happy. But give her space, give her time and give her help when she needs it. When we were walking down to the toilet, she was quite happy to talk then.'

Conclusions

Josephine was new to the unit. She was settling into the unit and would have preferred to have been going home. Josephine and Andrew had no previous experience of one another. What happened was their first encounter and it was free to be whatever it was going to be.

Andrew had been told that Josephine was anxious about her ankle ulcers, so he talked a fair amount while he tended the dressing, in order to allay her fears. He realised that she was not as concerned about her ulcers as he had been led to believe and that the ulcers were really a 'non-issue' for Josephine. He did the dressing carefully and helped Josephine walk to the toilet afterwards, still affirming with her that she was improving.

He felt that the main issue with Josephine was that she wanted to go home. He had been told that she had been 'negative' about being in the nursing unit and he thought this was reasonable, because she did not have to like being there. He gave her the right to feel as she wanted to feel.

Josephine was being herself, that is, she was being as she felt in that moment. The ulcers on her feet were inconsequential to her feeling tired and ready to go home. She knew that her walking was not stable when she was tired, so she realised that this was keeping her in hospital. She was not involved with the interaction with Andrew at first, and she appeared to be uninterested in the dressing of her ulcers. Towards the end of the interaction, however, she became more involved in what was going on, when she participated in the conversation and smiled occasionally at comments Andrew was making.

Josephine was getting to know Andrew. Although he was her primary nurse, he was a relative stranger at that point of their relationship, and it was reasonable to expect that she would not be forthcoming with comments and general involvement, if that was how she generally interpreted situations similar to this. As they walked to the toilet later, she offered comments freely. It took some time to begin to get to know one another.

Home was important for Josephine, but her desire to go home was not something she talked about freely. For her it almost went without saying that: 'Everyone likes being in their own home.' Whilst this statement may be one with which many people might identify, it was nevertheless a very strong statement about where Josephine was happiest to be, that is, in her own home. It doesn't matter how nice a hospitalised experience is, it is still not home, where you can be free to be yourself.

Researcher's postscript. Josephine said at the end of the conversation between us that she enjoyed the chat, to which I registered surprise. I made some notes in my journal that: 'I registered genuine surprise here, given that the interaction had seemed to me to be fairly 'flat' throughout' and in response to Josephine saying: 'A little chat with anybody is always nice,' I reflected that:

> 'She has appreciated chatting. Could it be that the chatting helped to make the difference towards the end of the interaction, when she chatted with Andrew, and then later, in our talk together? Going home is important, but it seems that chatting is also.'

Time was helpful in seeing my own involvement in this interaction. I realised that I had certain expectations about how the interaction might have been, and that I now find that it was as it was, because Andrew and Josephine accepted each other as they were, as a nurse doing a careful job, and as a patient feeling ready to go home.

4. Elizabeth's nurse-patient interactions

Introducing Elizabeth

Elizabeth was in her early twenties, when she began her nurse training in 1960. She became a nurse because she had been a patient and she was impressed by the care she received. She likes Virginia Henderson's definition of nursing, that nurses do things for people that they would do for themselves if they were in a well enough state. Elizabeth likes nursing, because of the patient contact and the satisfaction she derives from helping people. Since these stories of nursing care, Elizabeth has taken up a new job as an assessment nurse for a geriatric assessment team. She enjoys community nursing and working with a multidisciplinary team. Elizabeth hopes that nursing in the future will become more autonomous, considering different things that people might have in their health care, such as alternative therapies, if they want them.

Introducing Coralina

Coralina was born 28 October 1905. She lives at home with her unmarried son. Coralina was admitted to hospital for a laparotomy, after which she developed congestive cardiac failure and pulmonary oedema. She recovered for some time in the Intensive Care Unit, before being transferred to a general ward. Eventually, Coralina was transferred to the Professorial Nursing Unit for rehabilitation, with the aim of making her as self-sufficient as possible. Coralina is now able to do most things to help herself with her activities of daily living, but her feet are swollen, and her legs are weak, and some dyspnoea persists; thus walking is difficult.

Elizabeth and Coralina: a story about a shower and change of clothes

Coralina is already in the shower. I realise that Elizabeth is with her as I make a bed with Andrew. I go to them and remind Elizabeth that Coralina has given permission for me to be there. She nods. I remind Coralina of our conversation of yesterday. She remembers. I tell Elizabeth I will stand back out of the way. When I offer to help her if she thinks she needs me, Elizabeth says that Coralina prefers to have only one person with her.

The shower room is narrow, enclosed in tiled walls on two sides, with a frosted window behind the shower taps. It is very warm in the room. I stand out of the immediate area, beyond the activity between Elizabeth and Coralina. I want to keep out of the way, yet see and hear what I can to understand what is happening.

Coralina has finished the washing part of her shower and is beginning to dry her body. She is a large, strong looking, German woman of heavy build. Her face is soft and plump, her cheeks are full, and her skin is smooth and wrinkled at the edges of her round countenance. Her hair is grey and cut short, hanging presently in wet tufts around her face. Her neck is slightly flexed, orienting her face downwards towards her chest. She is almost naked, covered in part by a towel.

Elizabeth is wearing a white shirt and navy blue skirt, which shows traces of talcum powder from previous engagements in the shower room this morning. On her feet she wears protective plastic covers. She is intent on assisting Coralina. They are wiping Coralina's body together. 'What part haven't you done?' asks Elizabeth. 'Have you dried your bosoms?' Coralina takes the towel and dries under and around her breasts. Elizabeth waits while Coralina helps herself. For each part of Coralina's body to be dried, there is encouragement and praise from Elizabeth, who waits to allow her to be as independent as possible.

There is not much room at the end of the narrow shower space. Coralina is sitting on a shower chair and Elizabeth is standing in front of her. The room remains warm and feels closed in. I notice that the floor at the entrance to the shower cubicle near where I am standing, has a slight downhill angle, which has been fashioned in a ramp shape to allow wheelchair access. I wonder how the angle affects people with wet feet, and how wheelchairs fare with misapplied brakes. My attention returns to Elizabeth and Coralina.

As much of the exposed parts of Coralina's body as is possible have been dried. 'Now we are ready to put your clothes on,' announces Elizabeth. Elizabeth walks to the outside of the room and takes each piece of clothing in turn from off the back of the wheelchair, where it has been hanging. Coralina's pants go on first. Elizabeth bends down to put them on. Coralina helps by lifting her feet and legs a little. The pants stay near the top of Coralina's knees for the time being. Elizabeth hands Coralina her petticoat and leaves her for a few seconds to get the next piece of clothing. Coralina realises it is turned the wrong way, so she turns it in the correct way, before she puts the petticoat on over her head and pulls it down.

Elizabeth returns and praises her for putting the slip on herself. Coralina smiles. Coralina's smile is like a sunbeam sweeping suddenly across a shadowy plain. Coralina's smiles come when she is amused by what Elizabeth is saying, or when she is pleased with the way in which she is being praised for her efforts.

'This is a lovely pink colour. Do you like it?' says Elizabeth as she raises Coralina's frock to put it over Coralina's head. 'Yes,' replies Coralina. Her voice is thick and abrupt. Coralina is not saying much more that a few words at a time. Her first language is German, but she is also puffing with the effort of getting dried and dressed, and she is attending to what must be done to get her ready.

It is time to stand up. Elizabeth is at Coralina's side telling her what to do. Elizabeth leans forward in the chair and tries to stand up to lean over the wheelchair, which Elizabeth has placed in front of Coralina, but the first few attempts are fruitless and Coralina begins to say that she cannot do it. Elizabeth says that it might be the towel slipping under her feet, so she removes it from under Coralina's swollen feet. Elizabeth encourages her to try again and tells her to press down on the arms of the shower chair, in which she is sitting. Coralina tries again and lifts herself slowly upward and forward. Elizabeth does not rush her. She allows Coralina to do it herself, in her own time.

Coralina leans forward and Elizabeth tells her she is drying her bottom and then Elizabeth pulls up Coralina's pants, which have been waiting 'half-mast' at her knees. 'Now stand up straight,' says Elizabeth softly but firmly. 'Put your arms out here,' indicating the side-rails on the walls of the cubicle. Coralina stretches herself slowly to full height. 'That's the hard part over,' says Elizabeth. 'Now for the easy bit. All you have to do now is turn around and sit down.' Moving her hands carefully on the side-rails, Coralina turns and eases herself slowly into the waiting wheelchair. I think about the incline at the entrance to the shower cubicle, not far from the back wheels of the chair, but Elizabeth has the brakes on firmly and she moves around the back of the wheelchair as Coralina settles herself.

It's time for teeth cleaning. Coralina has moved in her wheelchair to the hand basin. Coralina cleans her dentures with care at the hand basin, whilst Elizabeth waits quietly at her side. When she has almost finished, Elizabeth tells Coralina that she has done an extremely good job. 'Not so good!' gruffs Coralina. 'No, I think you were very good,' assures Elizabeth. Coralina does not argue, but finishes off cleaning her dentures. She settles back in the chair, smiling, as Elizabeth wheels her out towards her bed.

'You carry the bowl,' Elizabeth says, handing Coralina the wash bowl carrying the toiletries. Coralina rests it in her lap. I have a sense of 'That's phase one finished!' It is time now for a foot massage. Back at the bed, Elizabeth puts away the shower things and sits down on a stool at Coralina's feet. She rubs peanut oil into her feet, right foot first, as the doctor enters. Elizabeth looks up and tells him the massage will strengthen Coralina's feet and keeps on massaging as he talks with Coralina. Elizabeth tells the doctor that Coralina is trying very hard to manage by herself as much as possible. He tells Coralina that she can go home on Friday night to see how she can manage with whatever support she has at home.

The doctor says Coralina will need to see how she can do things like getting herself into and out of bed. Coralina says, with a smile, that her son at home is strong. We laugh and the doctor says 'Yes, but he may not always be there. We will see how you go.' She is keen to go home, she says so when the doctor asks if this is what she really wants. Coralina is watching Elizabeth at her feet as she responds in single words to the doctor. The conversation is about the importance of trying to do things herself and co-operating with helpers. Elizabeth says that Coralina can be fairly frightening to her helpers at times and looks at her and says with a smile, 'You frighten me sometimes when you growl at me!' 'I am a gentle woman. I don't frighten anyone!' Coralina booms quickly, and then adds, 'Sometimes!' That smile sweeps over her face again, a smile to melt snow in winter.

Interpretations

Using the method of analysis discussed previously in Chapter 2, six main qualities and activities emerged from the text relating to the interaction between Elizabeth and Coralina, which appeared to illuminate the phenomenon of ordinariness in nursing. The qualities and activities were: approving commendable human qualities; valuing the importance of home; expressing feelings; expressing affection and liking; relating to the other's situation and enjoying a sense of humour.

Approving commendable human qualities. Coralina expressed her appreciation of the qualities she admired about Elizabeth, most of which were connected to the ways in which she helped Coralina. She said of Elizabeth:

> 'Washed me the back, help me when I need something to give me. She's very nice...She help all she can. She help me wash the back, the feet where I not can. Only in the front I wash self...She's alright, alright...She helps you, she's nice, she makes you comfortable.'

Of the other nurses, Coralina said:

> 'They are lovely. They do what they can.'

Valuing the importance of home. Coralina had been home on 'weekend leave.' Coralina's son, Peter, had been there to help her and they were able to converse in their first language. Coralina said:

> 'On the weekend I was home, I lie on the bed and watch the television. We talk and talk. It was lovely.'

She acknowledged how much she relied on her son to help her.

> 'I cannot (do much). Peter must help or I lie there. I can do nothing.'

Coralina hoped she would be able to go home to stay, although she was concerned that ultimately she would not be able to manage.

> 'Yes. Yeah. I happy when I come home...Some time it's very hard. You like home again. You like home...At weekend I go home again.'

Elizabeth knew how important Coralina's son was to her recovery, but she was cautious about using the strategy he had 'license' to use with her to motivate her. Elizabeth explained:

> 'Her [Coralina's] son uses a different approach. He feels he's got to make her angry to get her to do anything. That's what he said to us: "She won't do anything unless you make her angry." So when the others tried that...I wasn't told this, and that's not my way anyway. I can't use confrontation to make people do things. I don't think it works. Some of the others did, and she just doesn't have a good relationship with the ones that made her angry...She knows that he [Coralina's son] really cares anyway...Yeah. It didn't work, she was not doing a thing. I came into the picture when she'd been admitted a few days. I'd been away, and they were saying: "There's a stubborn old lady who wouldn't move, who had to be lifted everywhere." Within half a day she was doing these things for herself.'

Expressing feelings. As Coralina continued to talk about going home, she expressed her fear that her rehabilitation might not be successful and it might be better to go the a nursing home. Coralina said:

'Yes. I do what I can. I only wish sometime.' [Coralina began to cry]...I wish [spoken in German]...When you think, sometime I think it's been a long time I lie here, I much rather [a nursing home]. I don't know.'

Elizabeth expressed her sadness at the fairly likely inevitability of Coralina needing to be cared for in a nursing home.

'I think she'll probably be alright for a little while, but I think eventually she's going to be too much for the family to look after. I think that's really sad, but a little way down the track, she'll probably have to go to a nursing home...Oh yeah. She has improved a lot. I think there's a limit to the amount of improvement she'll show.'

Coralina and Elizabeth were able to express their feelings about how Coralina felt about trying to help herself, and how she was trying to improve her attempts at independence. Elizabeth explained how she succeeded, where other nurses failed, to motivate Coralina.

'I don't know really. She [Coralina] gave me a big cuddle when she saw me and I said: "How difficult it must be for you to be in this situation," and she was a bit teary and she gave me a cuddle, and said: "Yeah." I said: "I'm sure we can work out a way that we can do it better than this." So we talked about it. I said: "Maybe we could give some massage to your legs and maybe that would give you a bit more strength." I don't think it does actually. I think it's psychological.'

Expressing affection and liking. Elizabeth explained how she had come to know Coralina and the liking that had developed between them.

'I feel it's a good time, having a shower, to build up a positive relationship, which I feel I've got with Coralina. Right from the first time we met, she seemed to take a shine to me and would try harder for me than she would for the others for some reason. I don't know why. Doing intimate things with her helps us to get a bit closer. She needs to feel that somebody cares before she'll do something, really. It's a nice sort of way to show that you care. I think touching her, she enjoys touch, and she gets comfort from that. She responds nicely. She also likes her feet massaged and she feels that that gives her more strength, so she can stand more easily.'

Relating to the other's situation. Elizabeth knew Coralina for some time, during which time, using a number of subtle cues, she related to how Coralina was feeling at various occasions.

'Sometimes she really is too tired and you can tell. You don't push her. I don't push her. I just let her go at her own pace. You can tell by her tone of voice and her body language if she's really had enough, and so you can call it quits then. I think it's just a combination of things; the way she says things, her body language and whether she really looks tired. Yeah, I think we do get to know our patients pretty well. Especially having the same patient the whole time.'

Enjoying a sense of humour. Coralina had a sense of humour; it emerged from time to time and lit up her face with a radiant smile. Sometimes Coralina's smile would come in response to Elizabeth's praise or gentle persuasion.

I wrote these notes about Elizabeth helping Coralina in the shower.

Elizabeth returns and praises her for putting the slip on herself. Coralina smiles. Coralina's smiles come when she is amused by what Elizabeth is saying or pleased with the way in which she is being praised for her efforts.

As an adjunct to her own words, these notes are about a conversation between a doctor, Coralina, and Elizabeth.

Elizabeth says that Coralina can be fairly frightening to her helpers at times and looks at her and says with a smile 'You frighten me sometimes when you growl at me!' 'I am a gentle woman. I don't frighten anyone!' Coralina booms quickly and then adds 'Sometimes!' That smile sweeps over Coralina's face again; a smile to melt snow in winter.

Conclusions

Coralina was a large German woman, who appeared gruff and stubborn, but who was as soft as her smile and was waiting to be treated sensitively. Her breathlessness and her swollen feet made walking impossible for her and she was glad of the independence her wheelchair gave her. She tried to help herself as much as possible, but she despaired that, ultimately, she would be unable to care for herself.

When Coralina was first admitted to the PNU she gained a reputation for being slow to help herself. Coralina's son passed on his ideas to the nurses in good faith, but he failed to realise that what works between his mother and himself, may not work with relative strangers. As a matter of personal preference, Elizabeth chose to disregard the son's advice to make Coralina angry, to get her to do things for herself. Elizabeth knew the difference in what Coralina would accept as motivational strategies from her son and from the nursing staff. Elizabeth felt that family members have special licence with one another, and that understanding between family members is built up over a lifetime. This is not so with strangers, however well intentioned their actions.

Elizabeth preferred to take things gently with Coralina and to talk with her about what Coralina thought she could do and how Elizabeth could help her to do it. Coralina and Elizabeth took time to get to know one another and to talk about it together. They worked together, rather than following the previous approaches which were designed to work on Coralina rather than with her. Coralina cuddled Elizabeth, who expressed her understanding of Coralina's plight. The result was a special relationship in which Coralina tried to help herself and Elizabeth gave her respect and encouragement. The relationship between Coralina and Elizabeth was effective, because they treated each other sensitively as unique human beings.

Coralina was despondent about the time it was taking for her to recover. Coralina suspected that she needed to go to a nursing home, although she preferred to go home to be with her son. She mentioned that her son was strong and that he was at home, as she recounted the lovely time they had together, when she was at home for the weekend recently. Home was the preferred place for Coralina, but she feared she would not be able to stay there. Elizabeth felt sorry that Coralina might have to go to a nursing home. She knew Coralina's capabilities; they planned Coralina's independence together, but Elizabeth knew that there was only so much Coralina could do to help herself. Elizabeth felt for Coralina, knowing that she would rather be at home, but that she may end up in a nursing home ultimately. Coralina's destiny mattered to Elizabeth.

Coralina appreciated Elizabeth because she helped her as much as she needed it and she was nice to her and made her comfortable. It was important for Coralina that nurses helped her and that they were nice to her. In the world of the PNU something as simple as niceness and comfort could bring a smile to a seemingly 'gruff and stubborn' German woman, who would have loved to have been going home to stay.

Introducing Joe

Joe was born on 16 November 1921. He lives at home with his wife. Joe was admitted to hospital for the surgical insertion of a dynamic hip screw into his right fractured femur and was transferred to the PNU for rehabilitation. He is beginning to ambulate and to resume his activities of daily living.

Elizabeth and Joe: a story about feeling at home in a professional setting

I walk with Elizabeth to Joe's bed. It is in a large rectangular room opening onto a sunroom, which houses seven beds in several partitions. Joe is sitting on a chair beside his bed. He is reading a newspaper and drinking a stubby of beer. He is dressed in his house clothes and looks fresh and clean after his shower. The ward is noisy. People are talking and a child is crying loudly.

Elizabeth tells him she would like to look at the dressing on his right ankle and she suggests he might like to get himself into bed, to demonstrate what he learned with the occupational therapists this morning. Joe says he wasn't very successful this morning, as he pulls himself up the bed a bit higher and tries to put his foot under his right leg to ease it onto the bed. He makes several attempts, before Elizabeth helps him onto the bed.

She positions him comfortably and tells him she will take the dressing off. Joe tells her the pain he experienced in the ankle this morning kept him awake for several hours. She takes the dressing off carefully and finds that there is new skin over the wound and that it is healing nicely. She palpates around the perimeter of the wound and asks him to tell her when it feels sore. He indicates a sore spot and she bends down to have a closer look and to give the area a gentle rub.

She says she will go and prepare a dressing for it, that is to be left on for about four more days, at which time, she predicts, it will be healed. While she is away, Joe tells me that he enjoyed his shower given to him by a student nurse this morning, and that I should pass the word on to the student's teachers that she did a thoroughly good job.

When Elizabeth returns she brings the student nurse back with her to show her the dressing and Joe nods to me: 'She's the one' he mouths. I nod that I understand. Joe knows that I am from the university faculty and that the nurse is in the preregistration course there. Elizabeth explains the status of the wound and the purpose of the dressing to the nurse and then demonstrates to her how the new dressing is applied. Joe is lying quietly with his eyes shut and only opens them when they have finished. Elizabeth reminds him of how long the dressing will need to stay on.

She suggests he might like to get out of bed and Joe manages to get himself out, quipping that it's easier to get out than to get in. The student nurse brings the frame to him and he stands upright, before moving towards his chair a few steps away. Elizabeth suggests that he might like to go for a walk and the nurse consults her wrist watch and agrees. 'Be buggered I will!' he exclaims, and begins to tell them that he walked this morning. The student nurse says that it was an hour ago, and he disagrees looking at Elizabeth and telling her with a grin that 'This one is a slave driver!' The student nurse and Elizabeth give in to Joe's resistance to go walking again and he lets himself down in his chair.

Elizabeth and the student nurse stand beside him a while, and Elizabeth suggests that Joe could have a massage from the student nurse, and then Elizabeth looks at her and says she thinks it would be good if she could have one herself right now, because she has had a stiff neck. They both walk to a spare chair, which is situated between Joe's bed and the window, and Elizabeth sits down. The student nurse begins to massage Elizabeth's neck and she shuts her eyes with relief.

Joe looks over to them and says that it looks like Elizabeth is going to sleep. He smiles and turns his attention to his beer and his paper. The massage continues for about five more minutes, with Joe involving himself in their conversation from time to time. The noise in the ward has abated slightly. The child has stopped crying and is now talking. I go to Joe and thank him for allowing me to be there and ask him whether he'd like to talk with me after lunch, and before he goes to physiotherapy, and he thinks that is a good idea.

Interpretations

Joe was recovering after surgical treatment for his fractured femur. He was becoming able increasingly to ambulate and he was pleased to receive any help the nurses gave him. In this interaction, Elizabeth attended to Joe's ulcer dressing on his heel, because it had been causing him pain and he had had a restless night.

When I analysed the text relating to the interaction between Elizabeth and Joe, I located eight main qualities and activities, which appeared to illuminate the phenomenon of ordinariness in nursing. The qualities and activities were: approving commendable human qualities; appreciating skilful nursing care; appreciating help; tolerating noisiness; appreciating a 'home-like' atmosphere; relating to one another's humanness; talking 'straight'; and expressing feelings. These qualities and activities will now be described.

Approving commendable human qualities. Joe was appreciative of Elizabeth, and of the nurses generally. Of Elizabeth he said:

> *'She was very attentive and very nice, yes.'*

Of the other nurses Joe said:

> *'I don't think I can think of anything else to say, bar that the nurses are lovely.'*

Appreciating skilful nursing care. Joe appreciated the way in which Elizabeth tended his dressing and made him comfortable. He explained:

> *'It [the dressing procedure] was very pleasant, actually...because I had pain throughout the night and I wanted it. You always appreciate the things that they do for you. She [Elizabeth] turned me over on my side and put a pillow between my legs and made me comfortable.'*

Appreciating help. Joe was appreciative of any help the nurses gave him. He said:

> *'They are very helpful and they look after you real well. I can't say enough for them.'*

Joe was also appreciative of the way in which he was learning to help himself.

> *'Yes, because I've gotta learn to do it. Yes, it is important to me. That's what I mean. They will help when you want help. They'll let you do what you can yourself, but if they find you can't do it, they'll help you.'*

Tolerating noisiness. The noise level in the ward was noticeably high, during Elizabeth's and Joe's interaction. Elizabeth related to her tolerance for noisiness to a 'home-like' atmosphere and Joe seemed to take comfort in the noise. Noise and homeliness seemed to co-exist in the unit. Joe said he did not mind the noise in the ward and put forward his reason why.

> *'[The noise is] quite comfortable. They are all very nice people, the nurses and everything like that!'*

Elizabeth did not notice the noisiness of the ward. She said:

> 'No, I didn't notice...Well, when you've brought up two children you learn to 'cut off.'

Appreciating a 'home-like' atmosphere. Joe felt that the unit was like home. He said:

*'Oh, they treat you like you're at home, I think myself...Fixing your
meals up and showering and they help you every way they possibly can.'*

Elizabeth realised that when she had a massage at Joe's bedside
that it was a natural thing to do and that Joe appreciated the friendly
atmosphere it facilitated. Elizabeth explained:

'Yes, well, I needed one [a massage]. [Laugh] But, I thought
afterwards that Joe liked the friendly atmosphere, just like you do
at a friend's house. I think here [in the PNU] they [the patients]
treat us more as friends and equals, than they do on other
wards...Yes. I think he felt comfortable in the situation.'

Expressing feelings. Elizabeth acknowledged Joe's anxiety about
his painful heel.

'He was very anxious about his heel, because he has had trouble
with it for the past two years, he tells me. He has had skin grafts
and pressure sores, that developed after a hip replacement was done.
So, being aware of his anxiety, I decided to take down the dressing,
even though it wasn't time. I decided to take the Duoderm [wound
application] off. There was no indication that there was anything
going on underneath, apart from that he needed to be reassured
that it was OK. I took down the dressing. It was fine. It seemed to
put his mind at ease, because the pain seemed to disappear, once
he realised that there was no problem.'

Relating to one another's humanness. Elizabeth believed that
people should be encouraged to do things at their own pace and to
do what they are capable of at any particular point in time. Elizabeth
explained:

'I don't believe in pushing them too far. They will only do what
they are able to do. If you push them, they will only do less or
when you are there. If they have the motivation to do it, they'll do
it when you are not there as well.'

Talking straight. Joe felt quite within his rights to talk straight.
Joe managed to speak plainly about how he saw things, at the same
time maintaining a sense of humour. I recounted the episode in
my journal in this way:

'She suggests he (Joe) might like to get out of bed and Joe
manages to get himself out, quipping that it's easier to get out
than get in. The student nurse brings the frame to him and he
stands upright before moving towards his chair a few steps away.
Elizabeth suggests he might like to go for a walk and the nurse
consults her watch and agrees. "Be buggered I will!" he exclaims
and begins to tell them that he walked this morning. The student

nurse says that it was an hour ago and he disagrees looking at Elizabeth and telling her with a grin that "This one is a slave driver!" The student nurse gives in to Joe's resistance to go walking again and he lets himself down in his chair.'

Elizabeth interpreted this exclamation by saying:

'Yes. He stuck up for himself!'

Conclusions

Joe was getting stronger and he was thankful for the help Elizabeth gave him. He was also appreciative of the student nurse's care and he commended her to me and to her teachers. Joe appreciated nurses helping him. Even though helping was an expected part of a nurse's role, it rated a mention with Joe.

Joe had been experiencing pain overnight. Elizabeth took Joe's pain seriously and found his anxiety ample reason for attending to his dressing. She reassured him that the wound was OK. She connected his discomfort to anxiety and she acknowledged his anxiety as a legitimate reason for doing his dressing. After Elizabeth tended the dressing, Joe was contented that there was nothing wrong under his ankle dressing.

Elizabeth demonstrated the dressing technique to a student nurse and involved her in Joe's ongoing care by suggesting a walk. Joe refused to do further walking, because he felt he had done enough for a while. He defended himself by straight talking in a jovial way, because he knew he had the right and opportunity to speak up for himself and he knew that he would be heard. Joe's unwillingness to do further walking was judged as reasonable by Elizabeth and the student nurse.

Elizabeth suggested that the student give Joe a massage, but before Joe responded, Elizabeth decided she needed one herself. It was quite natural for Elizabeth and the nurse to take up their positions at the side of Joe's bed to massage Elizabeth's neck. Elizabeth attributed her own willingness to sit and be massaged, to the shared understanding of the rights of nurses and patients as 'friends and equals' in the unit. In this environment it was reasonable to acknowledge her own needs, even though she was 'at work'.

Elizabeth was pleased that what was natural and helpful for her to do, was also enjoyable for Joe. She noticed Joe enjoyed being a part of the massage and felt that it created a homely atmosphere.

Joe enjoyed watching Elizabeth have her massage and he involved himself in a companionable sort of way. He continued to drink his beer and read his paper, giving a comment here and there, much as one would do in a comfortable, home-like place.

Joe was comfortable in all the noise of the relatively open ward, because of the care he received, and because of the homely way in which the unit was conducted. It didn't matter to Joe that the geographical features of the room caused noise to carry because, for him, the people made it worthwhile. He equated the nursing care with home. He felt that he was being looked after as well as if he were at home. It wasn't just that it was like home in the unit, from the point of view of being helped, but it also had to do with what he was reasonably expected to do for himself.

Elizabeth was not aware of the noise levels in the room during her interaction with Joe. Elizabeth was no stranger to noise, given her previous home experiences as a mother of two children. There was a certain 'homeliness' in the ward noise, which Joe and Elizabeth accepted as part of the context. In this interaction the noise and bustle did not matter, because there was a comfortable rapport existing between them, in which they gave each other freedom to be 'friends and equals.'

Introducing John

John was born on 12 February 1936. He lives on a ten acre farmlet with his wife. John is an ex-butcher, of Hungarian descent. He has insulin dependent diabetes mellitus and has been admitted to the PNU for stabilisation of his blood sugar levels.

Elizabeth and John: a story about trying to eat sensibly

John is unpacking his things, just after he is admitted to the unit. He is a short, stout man, wearing blue trousers and a tee shirt pulled firmly around his round abdomen. His broad, open face is tanned and his ready smile reveals a gap in his teeth, making his appearance friendly and somewhat 'cheeky.' He has a greying moustache and eyebrows and his grey hair is short and tidy.

After the usual explanations, John agrees to be in my research project, so I thank him and I tell him I will be back when Elizabeth comes to talk with him. I return later to John's bed and I realise from his file on the bed, that Elizabeth is not far away. I find a seat as Elizabeth enters and I sit on the opposite side of the bed to her and John. She pulls up a chair to face him. They are both near a window, which has the curtain drawn. John is sitting in front of the bedside locker.

Elizabeth begins by telling him about the unit, how it is relaxed and as homely as possible. She tells him that nurses are not in uniform here, but rather they are in their 'street clothes'. As far as possible, he should try to keep all the routines he enjoys at home and he can make himself a tea or coffee when he likes. She tells him that the continuation of his home routines does not apply to eating whatever he likes though, and they smile together. She asks him about his routines at home, when he takes his insulin, when he likes to shower and go to bed, and so on. Elizabeth asks John to tell her why the doctor has sent him into hospital and they begin to discuss his diabetes.

He says his blood sugars are high and that he feels OK. He says his urine test was one quarter percent this morning and Elizabeth asks him whether it was the first urine after sleeping. When he says that it was, she explains that the first urine has been accumulating in the bladder overnight and the result may not always be accurate. He says he has a high blood pressure and cholesterol level and that the doctor is also worried about the circulation in his feet and that sometimes his soles feel like they are burning. When they begin to talk about his diabetes treatment, he says he loves to eat and finds it difficult to stay on a diabetic diet. Whenever he makes a confession, he smiles.

John says he gave up smoking three years ago on the day of his middle daughter's twenty-first birthday. He beams and pats his pockets as he describes how he sometimes looks for a smoke when he is anxious or angry. He remembers to the day when he stopped smoking, because of its association with his daughter's birthday. He speaks of his daughters frequently, but only of his wife when Elizabeth asks.

John's wife has leg ulcers and it seems that she does not play an active part in the domestic duties. John says that he does most of the cooking and lists the food he enjoys most. Having retired from being a butcher six years ago, he confesses a love for meat and says that he loves to make soup out of bones. Elizabeth explains that soup is fine if he lets it cool and skims the fat off the top, but he thinks she means he should eat it cold, so they take some time to clear up his misconception. I think how hard it must be for people like John to keep on a diet, especially when he loves food so much and is imaginative in cooking it.

Elizabeth suggests that they go on a tour of the unit, so I thank them both very much for allowing me to attend their interaction and say that I will catch up with them soon.

Interpretations

John was a retired butcher, who loved to eat. He had been admitted to the PNU to assist in the stabilisation of his insulin dosage, in order to manage his diabetes. John was aware of the theory of diabetes management, but he seemed unable to put that knowledge into practice in his own life. In this interaction, Elizabeth admitted him to the nursing unit and began to build a friendly relationship with him.

I found seven main qualities and activities when I analysed the text relating to the interaction between Elizabeth and John, and they were: acknowledging the importance of company and talking; valuing the importance of home; appreciating a 'home-like' atmosphere; acknowledging the relevance of family affiliations; facilitating coping; tolerating one another's humanness; and relating to the other's situation. These will be discussed in the section that follows.

Acknowledging the importance of company and talking. John appreciated the time Elizabeth took with him on his admission to the unit, to explain about the set up of the place and what to expect in relation to his nursing and medical care. John said:

> 'Yes I did [enjoy the chat with Elizabeth], because it was so friendly …Everything was perfect…She made it clear what I had to do and how this place is different…Actually it was special, because I never had treatment in the hospital like that before…Was very good. [It was the] first time [that] they [nurses] explain where you are, what you can do, the treatment you can do.'

Valuing the importance of home. For all the praise John heaped on the PNU, it was still less attractive than home. John explained:

> 'It is better to be home. I'm such a person, I can survive anywhere. Whatever I have to do. I listen to the person and whatever they tell me, I do it and no problems.'

Appreciating a 'home-like' atmosphere. John was impressed with the amount of freedom he had in the PNU to continue with his usual routines. He said of the unit:

> 'Good place…So far, I feel like it at home. Nobody push you around. In the morning, wake up at seven o'clock for insulin. I do it myself. For the last ten years, I can do it, so.'

Elizabeth noticed that John enjoyed the homeliness of the PNU
She said:

> 'He seems to have settled in really well and he is treating it like
> home. He thinks the homely atmosphere is nice. He feels free to
> come and go as he pleases. He is doing more exercise, which is
> good. He might continue it when he goes home.'

Acknowledging the relevance of family affiliations. John was
very keen to go home as soon as he could, because he had family
responsibilities. He said:

> *'I hope I can go home by Friday. My younger daughter go to Queensland
> on the weekend... If she goes then no-one can look after at home. My
> wife is not able to look after things, because of the leg. He [the doctor]
> says: "We will see what happens in three days." He says we might get
> home...That's what they told me last time and I was in nineteen days!'*
> *[Laugh]*

Facilitating coping. For John, the main reason for his hospitalisation was to learn to cope with his diabetes, especially in relation
to his diet.

> *'Yes. They are friendly and they teach you how you can cope at home
> and that's nice. Actually, that is all I want while I am here, how I can
> help myself.'*

Tolerating one another's humanness. Elizabeth was aware of
John's history of dietary noncompliance and she realised that he
knew what he should do, if he could find the willpower to do it.
She said:

> 'It was the first time I'd met him, but I read his history and he was
> a man who knew what he should be doing and he hadn't been
> doing it. I didn't want to put him on the spot, because many people
> have been on to him and it hasn't worked that way. I just tried to
> make it as informal as possible. He made a bit of a joke about his
> diet. He was quite amused by the fact that he likes his food and
> that's his trouble. I was trying to establish a friendly relationship.'

Relating to the other's situation. Elizabeth hoped that John
would benefit from relating to another patient's situation, by taking
up some of the advice he was giving to that person. She explained:

> 'He's learning how to do his blood sugars well. He is watching the
> education tapes. Every time you ask him something, he says: "But
> I already knew that! [laugh] but I don't do it." Interestingly, he's
> been having discussions with another man, who is a newly-
> diagnosed diabetic, who is in a quite anxious condition, and John
> is putting him at ease. He is teaching him a few things. So, maybe
> by advising this man, he may take his own advice.'

Conclusions

John loved to eat, but having diabetes made it difficult for him to be as spontaneous as he might like to be with his diet, without some problems arising from his high blood sugar levels. He was in the PNU to stabilise his insulin dosage. He knew what adequate compliance was in theory, because he told Elizabeth that the messages of the education tapes were familiar. He confessed to dietary indiscretions with a smile. He knew that what he needed most from the nurses was ways of how to cope at home.

Elizabeth did not judge and chastise John, as had been the approach of other health professionals. She noticed his sense of humour and his self-aware non-compliance and decided instead to work on building a friendly relationship. She knew he liked to eat and she realised he knew that his noncompliance was a problem. She knew he felt at home in the unit and she noticed he was exercising. She thought he might continue to exercise at home, but she made no value statements about his attitude towards compliance with treatment generally.

He appreciated the homely atmosphere in the unit and his freedom to feel a part of the place. He was encouraging a man who had been newly diagnosed as having diabetes, and the man was feeling some comfort from John's experience. Elizabeth was encouraged that John was helping another man with his diabetes education and she thought that it may help John to have helped someone else. She knew John knew the theory of diabetes management. She was hoping he would align more readily with adequate practice having encouraged someone else.

John's family was important to him and he was keen to go home, because his daughter was moving away and he needed to be at home to care for his wife. He knew that the nurses would be able to help him cope with how to manage his routines at home. As much as he appreciated the unit and the nurses in it, he would rather have been at home.

5. Jane's nurse-patient interactions

Introducing Jane

Jane always wanted to be a nurse, because she believed she could care for people. She began nursing 'at the very ripe old age of 36' and she has remained nursing for eight years. Jane thinks nursing is about treating a person as a person, and she cares for people in the way she would like to be cared for herself. Jane thinks 'a little bit of encouragement' is important in helping people to feel better. What Jane likes about nursing is knowing that she's helped someone, and what she doesn't like about nursing is the degree of medical dominance. Her hopes for nursing in the future, as an occupation going into the twentieth-first century, is that it will 'get back to its grass roots, the patient,' and put technology into perspective.

Introducing Ellen

Ellen was born 26 February 1904. She lives in a special accommodation nursing home, where she has her own shower and toilet facilities. Ellen was admitted to the Professorial Nursing Unit with a Colles fracture of her left arm, and a painful hip, which has since been diagnosed as a fracture of the left pubic ramus.

Jane and Ellen: a story about a wash in bed

Jane tells me she is ready to wash Ellen. Ellen will be resting in bed for a few days, because a fractured hip (mid pubis on the left side) has just been discovered on x-ray. This wasn't diagnosed when she was admitted. She has not had a fall since admission to the nursing unit, so it is a bit of a mystery as to how it happened.

We go to the bed and Jane tells Ellen why we are there. Jane is telling Ellen that she has a fractured hip and that it will be necessary for her to stay in bed for a while. Ellen is hard of hearing, so Jane sits close to her and has to repeat a few things to make sure Ellen

101

understands what she is saying. Ellen says she has a funny story to tell her and she looks at me and says: 'Do you think she's old enough to hear this?' I ask: 'Is nearly forty old enough?' She nods that it is. She tells us about a little girl and boy who go to a picnic and go behind a bush, because the little boy has to 'pee.' When the little girl sees 'what he has' she says: 'That's a handy thing to have on a picnic!' Jane gives Ellen a light tap on the arm as if to say 'Well, I never!' We all smile. Ellen says if she has to stay in bed it would be a handy thing for her to have, because it is much easier for males to manage when it comes to urination.

We begin to prepare for the wash by screening the bed and gathering the essentials. I go for a basin of water and clean towels, while Jane makes Ellen comfortable and covers her in a procedure wrap. As we begin to wash her, Jane talks to Ellen about the fracture of the hip and about the necessity to rest in bed. She asks how it happened and Ellen doesn't know. Jane prepares the washer and hands it to Ellen, who washes her face. When she has finished, I dry her face. When she washes her chest she says: 'I'd better wash under my flaps' and she lifts up her flattened breasts and washes under them. She instructs Jane to wipe under them as they recount together the first time Ellen referred to her breasts as 'flaps'. Ellen says Jane could not stop laughing and it has been their joke ever since. The washing, drying and talcing process continues until Ellen's body is freshened carefully.

As we work together, we talk. Ellen asks Jane where she comes from and whether she is an Australian. 'No, I'm from Birmingham, she says 'Or at least, that's what I tell people, because they know where that is. They wouldn't know the actual little place I come from.' 'I thought so,' says Ellen. 'I thought you were English; you have a good sense of humour.' Ellen tells us that she comes from the north of England.

The wash is over and Jane receives Ellen's teeth to take to wash them under running water. I pull the screens back and tidy the area. I find a comb and offer to comb Ellen's hair. As she moves her head forward, I also puff the pillow behind her. At this point, a doctor walks in and tells Jane she has a fractured hip, which wasn't there on admission, and asks her whether she has had a fall since being in hospital. She says 'Yes' at first, but she hasn't heard him properly. When he asks her again she confirms that she has not had a fall since admission. Another doctor and his 'understudy' walk in and begin to tell her the same thing, even though the former doctor tells them he has already told Ellen.

I exit with the wash bowl and towels just as Jane comes in and tells me Ellen's teeth are on the bench in the room opposite. I am pleased Jane is there with Ellen, because they are all talking at her and she is looking overwhelmed. I go to clean the teeth and when I return they have all gone and Ellen says: 'In this life we suffer grief and pain.' I listen, thinking that she wants to talk, but then she says: 'Would you hand me my beauty cream, please?' She applies some dabs of cream to her face and rubs them in. As I put the jar away she tells me it is Vitamin E and that usually she uses turtle oil. I ask her why she doesn't use it now and whether they have run out of turtles. She smiles softly at me.

Jane returns and apologises for getting caught up in the doctors' entourage. We adjust Ellen's bed to help her upright and Jane says that she will get something for her pain. Ellen draws Jane closer to her and looks in her eyes and says: 'I don't know what I'd do without you.' 'You'd manage,' Jane replies with a smile. But I wonder.

Interpretations

Using the method of analysis described previously in Chapter 2, I found five main qualities and activities in the text relating to the interaction between Jane and Ellen, which appeared to illuminate the phenomenon of ordinariness in nursing. The qualities and activities were: facilitating comfort; enjoying a sense of humour; relating to the other's situation; working competently; and needing continued help and attention.

Facilitating comfort. Ellen appreciated the wash Jane gave her, because it made her feel comfortable. Ellen said:

> 'Well, it [the wash] freshened me up and made me feel comfortable. I enjoyed it...I've got to be in bed and I've got to have my wash in bed, so I may as well enjoy it.'

Jane realised that Ellen's bedrest would require attention to her physical and mental comfort. She said:

> 'I don't know how I am going to cure her being bored. She can't knit because she has a fractured wrist and she can't hold the knitting. Her eyesight is not the best and her daughter said she might bring in some jigsaws. Later, she may be able to have a day out. I think once we can get her pain settled, now she knows why she has got the pain, that she will be OK.'

Enjoying a sense of humour. Humour was a strong bond between Ellen and Jane. Ellen enjoyed thoroughly Jane's sense of humour and Jane thought that Ellen was 'lovely' in the way she joked with her. Ellen felt that they were both cheeky and that was why she liked Jane so much. Ellen said:

> 'Yes, [I like her] because we are both cheeky. The other morning, the first morning I was in, I'd had my shower and I was trying to dress myself and I had a bit of trouble with my bra, so she [Jane] helped me and we got the bra on the front and the shoulder straps on and I said: "Now, wait a minute, I've got to get my flaps in yet." [laugh] You ask her! Well, [laugh] she said she had never heard anything like that. She was helping me put my bras on and a bit of powder and I said "Wait for my flaps," I said. Jane laughed, oh she laughed! She had to stop work for a while. You know, we get on sort of well. She's got a good sense of humour and I have…Oh well, she's such a happy person. I enjoy her. We have a joke when I have a wash. When I want a bit of powder on I put it on my wee flaps. The wash is a little bit of a joke, you know. She's a lovely girl, she is, a great sense of humour.'

On another occasion, Ellen demonstrated her sense of humour:

> 'Before I came down here, the night before, I was in bed and this young girl in the next bed and the nurse was sitting at the bottom. I had a lot of wind and I said "Oh, what's that noise!" Well, you should have heard this girl!'

Before she had her wash, Ellen shared a joke with us about the little girl and boy, who went on a picnic. Even so, Ellen claimed that she could not laugh and that she could not cry.

> 'But you know, I can't laugh. It is funny I can't laugh. I don't know. The only thing that makes me laugh is a [movie] picture, not a funny one, it's got to be a stupid one, a really stupid English one. Some pictures are just really stupid you know and I'll just laugh. I don't laugh and I don't cry…It seems that I just can't! Even when my husband was killed, I don't think I shed a tear.'

Jane enjoyed Ellen's sense of humour, to the point that she felt she had to explain that she was laughing with Ellen, not at her.

> 'Oh, honestly, she's lovely! I didn't quite know how to take her at first, because I thought she might be one of those whingeing old pommes, because some of them can be a real pain in the butt—so are many Australians! But she was really good. She said: "I need some help putting the bra on" and I sort of looked at it. She'd got it fastened before she'd even got into it! I said: "What are you doing that for?" "Well, this is how I did it yesterday," she said. "I fastened it and put it over my head like that and put it on by myself". I showed her another way of fastening it at the front and twisting it around. Well , she caught on and then all of a sudden, out of the blue, she said: "Well, now I'd better put my flaps in." I cracked up! Here she is, 87 years old, and she is gorgeous! She thought I was going to have a heart attack, I think. She said: "Well, what did

I say?" Normally they [older people] would be so staid. I apologised in the end. I said: "Look, I'm not laughing at you I'm laughing with you. I just think you are so gorgeous" Flaps! When we were making a bed later she said: "You tell that other Sister what I said!" She was really wrapped with this incident, so when she was having her ECG (electrocardiogram) done yesterday, she said to me: "I almost felt like saying to that girl when she was putting that cream on me, now mind my flaps!" I know it's going to get to the stage now when I'm helping to wash her where I say "Move your flaps" (laugh) It's is just so strange coming out of this 87 year old. After that incident I was with her in the afternoon and she said to me: "You know, you did me the world of good. It was good to have a laugh!" I thought that was good.'

Relating to the other's situation. Jane felt sorry for Ellen and for what each setback might mean for her.

'Yesterday she had a bit of a turn. She just said she felt like she was half awake, but she walked to the toilet and she got out and I said: "Do you want me to get a wheelchair?" and she said: "No, I'll be right" and, of course, one step and she staggered, and I said: "I'll get a wheelchair." Andrew brought the wheelchair down for me, so she went back to bed. Since then she has got further and further depressed I think. As much as I've tried to cheer her up and explain that it is only temporary and that she is going to get better, and we are going to make advances, but I feel so sorry for her because she just wants to get going.'

Working skilfully. Jane was a nurse with clinical knowledge and experience, which allowed her to practise nursing skilfully. Jane was suspicious of the pain Ellen experienced in her hip and pressed the matter with the doctors until the fracture was confirmed.

'Yesterday afternoon. She had really complained about the pain. I'd given her analgesics all day really to help her and I got a bit suspicious because it [the medical record] said "a painful right hip" and she was complaining about her left hip. Now, she's got bruising on the inner aspect of her right thigh and I thought, "Oh, yes, what's going on?" There was no mention of a fractured pelvic ramus [broken pelvic bone], so I thought I'd have a look at the x-ray results and it said that there was an undisplaced pelvic ramus. I thought I'd better get it looked into…They got the x-rays done and I was looking at them this morning [they weren't reported on] and I thought it looked a bit strange. It looked like she'd definitely done her pelvis, so I phoned the intern and told her I was inexperienced at reading an x-ray, but that it looked broken. She said she was as inexperienced as me in reading the x-ray, so I thought, "God!" She actually admitted that she couldn't read x-rays very well! She said she'd come up and we'd figure it out together. So up she comes, and by that time I'd looked at the first one and you could see the undisplaced part. So she took the x-rays straight away to have them confirmed and then they had a team meeting and came back and said that there was not much that they can do for it. I mean you can't put your pelvis together where that's broken. I thought they might have said to put her in pelvic girdle traction with weights to help get it in alignment...Her daughter was quite happy that we actually found out that there was something wrong. She thought that there was something wrong.'

Needing continued help and attention. Jane recognised Ellen's need for help and continued attention and hoped that she would be able to keep on being of use to her.

'It's just a matter of (Ellen) staying in bed now, and she's not a lady who likes staying in bed. She is just a bit miserable. But I think we got a few laughs...It's awfully hard talking to her, because she is deaf and sometimes I think she doesn't understand what she has been told or...I have said things to her and then she'll say to the next person: "What about such and such." It's a matter of keeping on repeating to her. She's down...I think she'll get there...I think that she does depend a lot on the personal touch. She likes to know that she's getting her little bit of attention. I just hope I can give it to her. I'd like to think that I've helped her.'

Conclusions

Ellen had just been told that she had a fractured hip and that she would have to stay in bed. She had been making progress, but the latest setback threatened to slow down her recovery and to keep her in hospital longer than she had anticipated. Ellen was discouraged about the enforced bedrest, but resigned herself to the verdict, saying that: 'While we are here, we suffer grief and pain.'

Ellen and Jane had a happy rapport, built on their collective sense of humour. They shared the joke about Ellen's 'flaps' and it has been their joke ever since. Ellen was delighted at Jane's wholehearted reaction and said Jane could not stop laughing. Ellen was pleased that she had amused Jane. It was interesting that Ellen claimed she couldn't laugh, which seemed incongruent in view of Jane's propensity to make her laugh, and the enjoyment she derived from making Jane laugh.

Ellen found commonalities in their national heritage and in their sense of humour. Ellen said to Jane: 'I thought you were English, you have a good sense of humour.' Ellen told us that she came from the north of England. Ellen liked Jane's sense of humour and she felt close to her, because she had a sense of fun.

Jane enjoyed Ellen's humour. She was surprised by Ellen calling her breasts her 'flaps' and she laughed so much, that she felt that she had to control herself and tell Ellen that she was laughing with her, not at her. She was afraid that she might have offended Ellen by laughing too much. Rather than be offended, Ellen was delighted with her laughter, and the incident became a theme, as a joke they shared together. The originality and placement of Ellen's humour was such a surprise that Jane discovered a common bond with Ellen, their love of humour, which transcended their respective circumstances and age differences.

Introducing Max

Max was born on 20 February 1949. When he was thirteen years old he experienced a cerebral subarachnoid haemorrhage. Four years later, after further neurological sequelae, he began to manifest signs of triplegia. Max lives at home with his mother, who supports him in looking after himself. He spends time in the local hospital whenever he has problems associated with immobility and he visits a large city hospital for assessment and rehabilitation as necessary. His most recent admission to the Professorial Nursing Unit was to allow healing of his sacral decubitis ulcer.

Jane and Max: a story about emptying a bowel

Jane tells me she is ready. We have just returned from morning tea together and she has decided that she will attend to Max now that we are back. She talks to me at the nurses' desk. She explains the gift box. It was given to her by the nursing staff at a party, because she has a reputation of being 'into this sort of stuff.' She opens the box. I see some writing on the outside. It looks like a quite usual gift box, but I sense it is not by the way Jane is smiling and going slightly flushed. 'I told Max I would present it to him today,' she says as she takes off the lid. Inside is a long coiled piece of plastic faeces on a bed of pink-coloured packing material. I laugh. We both laugh. 'Goodness, isn't it life like!,' I shriek.

We go to Max. Another nurse comes alongside, to see the presentation. Max smiles and shifts in the bed. 'I won't open it now' he says. Jane laughs lightly and leans into him. 'Oh yes you will!' she says. The other nurse agrees with the prompt and Max sneaks a quick look. He smiles broadly and leans back not talking, as we all enjoy a laugh together.

The other nurse leaves and we are left to get on with the procedure. Max tells Jane what she will need, things such as extra 'blueys,' (waterproof disposable sheets) a plastic bag, and so on. Although Jane and Max have a long history of being together in the previous PNU site, Jane has not yet done the procedure the 'new way,' which has been used since Max's last admission. Jane knows she will be pressing on his abdomen, whilst Max evacuates his bowel.

Jane goes off to get some more equipment and Max and I are left behind the curtain together. I notice his newly-arrived letter and suggest he'd probably have time to begin reading it while Jane is away. He says he won't bother. I notice his surname and ask him about his heritage. He tells me it is Swiss and I recount my only experience of Switzerland; how it looked like a chocolate box picture from the air. He tells me of his family who have lived in or visited Switzerland. Jane returns.

We set up the bed, protecting the linen and donning our plastic gloves. He is in the correct position, so Jane hands him a plastic glove and he puts it on his right hand. His hand goes down to his buttocks and he asks me if the dressing is out of the way. I am standing on that side and I tell him it is OK. There is silence. A few minutes later he says: 'I am just trying to locate my anus.' Jane nods.

Max tells Jane where to press on his abdomen and that the palpation he performed on himself earlier showed that he was not constipated. They talk together. Through the screens the sound of a radio opposite us is loud and cheerful, bopping along to a contemporary tune. We hear Hothouse Flowers sing 'I can see clearly now...' There are other sounds of movement and usual happenings outside the curtains, but in here, all is focussed on the job of getting faeces out of Max's bowel. I think about the flimsy barrier of curtain, the 'outside' and the 'inside' coexisting in a comfortable sort of way.

We are told that there is no faeces in the bowel. 'I'm trying to excite peristaltic action,' he says, in a casual, knowing sort of way. He is intelligent in so many ways. It is not just the knowledge of several medical terms, it is the quiet deliberance with which he goes about this task. He attends to his body as if he is in tune with its needs.

Jane says that he should tell her when he thinks he wants to give up and she waits quietly and patiently. He nods and continues to move his finger inside his anus. It is OK. He knows what is right for him. After about three more minutes, he decides that there is nothing there at all. Jane and Max discuss the causes of the empty bowel. Maybe his diet has been light. They recount the actual food he has eaten over the last few days. There is evidence of fibre in his diet. They agree that if the abdomen is not firm that it can be of little consequence that the evacuation is, for the time being, unsuccessful. They decide to leave a 'bluey' there just in case his bowel opens automatically later. 'That sometimes happens,' Jane says.

Max takes off his glove and we remove ours also. I offer to get the wash water, towels and washer, while Jane clears the area and makes ready for Max's wash. He tries to shift his body over to the side of the bed. He is thrashing about without a grip on the mattress. We both go to move forward. Jane says, as I think it: 'You will let me know if you want help?' He nods. I say that it is hard for me to hold back and allow him to help himself. Jane agrees. Max says that nurses interfering is not helpful. Jane explains to Max that she was trained to get in and do things and that now she is relearning how to help people, by letting them help themselves. She admits that she would like to help him, because he is struggling, and, beforehand, she would have thought it easier and quicker to intervene. He is lying still now, and he corrects her. He is not struggling. He is resting. She stands corrected.

He perseveres and on one last effort pushes himself up onto his left elbow. The effort of his thrust forward and upwards pushes some of the equipment on the overbed table. We hold onto it automatically, to save it from being propelled away from him. He says it is important for him to be independent. He demonstrates to us by his determination, just how important it is for him. The wash water, teeth cleaning bowls and towels are positioned. He will wash himself and push the buzzer when he wants us to come back. We go away. He buzzes for us in about half an hour.

When we enter the curtains, he is drinking directly from his water jug. Jane says that she thinks he should use a straw. Max says another nurse has told him that, as he continues to drink from the jug. Jane leaves to empty the wash water. He gulps down the last of the water and tells me that he should have an intake of at least two to three litres per day. Jane repeats that she thinks it looks awful to see anyone drinking directly from a jug. They exchange some words briefly about the aesthetics and practicalities of the habit and it is left unresolved, in as much as there is no assurance that it will not happen again, neither does Jane press him for such an undertaking. She has told him how it affects her, and that is enough.

The wash begins. We place the towels and begin the wash and dry Max's back, legs, groin and buttocks. At the point at which Jane is washing the scrotal area, they are having a discussion about a grazed area on the undersurface of the scrotal pouch. He admits that he caused it when he was turning himself. Jane is listening and responding to him. The music outside the curtain continues. Jane is looking intently at the scrotum, lifting carefully the folds to ensure a thorough wash, and painting lotion gently on the grazed area. The penis is washed with equal care and their conversation continues throughout. They could have been having this conversation in a sitting room, it is so comfortable and unselfconscious.

They exchange light banter, a word here, and a phrase there. It reflects their knowledge of one another. We all talk about Jane's daughter, as we complete the last touches of the wash. Max wonders what future she will have in primary school teaching. Jane explains that she is going to take a psychology major and have the chance to go into clinical psychology. I remark that schools provide excellent career counselling these days. The buttocks are washed and it is time for Max to roll over.

He lifts himself up onto his left elbow and turns his chest and body, as we guide his legs. He balances on both hands as we place a 'bluey' under his pelvic area. He is lying face down and we position the supporting pillows. Jane doesn't know which way the rubber square should be placed and says that it looks strange. He shows her the side which goes under his right leg and we position it carefully. He explains that the foam square helps to prevent skin loss when he has spasms and kicks out with that knee.

The top sheet is folded over at the top and left loose around his body. Jane comments on his hair and reminds him of the hair wash destined to happen later. 'I was hoping you would forget that,' he says with a smile. The area around the bed is quickly and thoroughly cleared away and Max is ready for lunch. Their conversation continues easily and is about what he would like placed next to him, how he feels now, what else he might need, all the time peppered with a smattering of lighthearted one-liner comments and jokes. His eyes are twinkling. He looks fresh and alert.

Interpretations

Max was bedridden with a slowly healing sacral bedsore. Ordinarily, he was able to move about in his wheelchair and be reasonably self sufficient, in spite of his triplegia. Jane knew Max as a patient and person, during his previous admissions to the unit, in which time she had maintained her care of him. On this particular occasion of nursing care, Jane and I gave Max some assistance with evacuating his bowel and with making him comfortable afterwards.

I analysed the text relating to the interaction between Jane and Max and six main qualities and activities emerged. The qualities and activities were: equating with a sense of 'that's all'; facilitating independence; enjoying a sense of fun; talking straight; relating to one another's humanness; and expressing feelings.

Equating with a sense of 'that's all'. Max tended to describe the procedure of bowel evacuation as nothing more than a task to be done, by people who knew what they were doing. He said:

> *'It's an everyday situation…Neither of us like doing it. We both know what has to be done, so it's not an embarrassment. Neither of us feel embarrassed by what's going on…I was just testing. I didn't have any funny feeling, that would mean that I would be constipated. I'm paralysed down there. With my hand I know what to look for and I knew I wasn't constipated. I put on a disposable glove and checked my lower bowel. It was completely empty. I could only find one wall of the bowel. There was nothing there. Nothing wanted to happen. The only thing that wanted to happen was that my sphincter muscle in my rectum was trying to push my finger out again. I kept it in there until I realised nothing was going to happen, so I let the sphincter muscle take over and quietly push my finger out and that was the end of it…We're both well aware that something may go wrong, but it won't phase us, that's all there is to it. It won't be embarrassing for either of us. It's just a procedure.'*

Max developed a sophisticated sense of independence, given the degree of his disability. When I commented that he did a good job of lifting himself onto his elbows, he said:

> *'It wasn't difficult [raising myself up onto my elbows]…Certain people are well aware that I haven't reached my maximum potential. I still haven't found out how far I can go…I'm just trying to retain maximum independence.'*

Facilitating independence. Max acknowledged that Jane allowed him to try to help himself. He gave an example of how he managed to raise himself onto his elbows.

> *'She [Jane] quietly lets me try my own techniques first before she intervenes. She would intervene at any time if something went wrong. The point is, I knew very well what she was worried about and I knew I was totally safe. If the top of the table snapped it wouldn't matter, because all I'd do is I'd fall back onto the bed.'*

Enjoying a sense of fun. Jane enjoyed the fun of the chocolate box presentation and knew that Max would be able to take the joke. Jane said:

'I couldn't resist that [presentation to Max], because that's something from his last stay with us. We had an Awards Night between the nurses and we all put in $5.00 and I got it back in the form of a piece of, (Oh, do I say it?)…a piece of fake shit. But when I was actually presented with it, it was saying that every Sunday and Wednesday I used to disappear [at work] for about half an hour and I'd always come back with a smile on my face, and so they all knew what I'd been doing. So because Max is a triplegic, he has to have 'manuals' [removal of faeces from the bowel] and everything, which he copes with himself at home. But they just made it as a huge joke. So to remember Max, I got this fake shit. So when he arrived, it was funny to see him again as a patient and I got told that he was back in, and I thought "Ah, my opportunity, I'll give it back to him!"…So I just presented it to him and I made him open the box, and the look on his face!!!…I can't describe this, but it was a look that I thought I was going to get.'

Talking straight. Jane and Max were accustomed to talking straight with each other. Jane explained:

'Because I think I know him really well, we've got a good rapport. I like him as a person. We call a spade a spade. We've had a few run-ins, in the first admission. I can sort of have a joke with him and he can tell me to shut my face or do whatever, and let me know it's not meant to be offensive or anything. Yet, I also think I know when it's time to back off.'

Jane gave an example of some straight talk, which went on between them both just after she returned from her holidays to find a different Max from the man she felt she knew.

'Later on in the afternoon I went to see him and asked him about his turn [pressure care]. He said: "Oh you do what you like" and I said: "Max I don't do what I like, I do what you want me to do." "Oh," he said, "the others do this that and the other" and I said: "Where's the fight gone Max?" and he started to cry and the first thing I did was put my arms around him, because I'm a tactile person. I know if people don't want to be touched. He didn't back off he didn't freeze or anything, he just laid there. He just started and said: "Well you know what drugs I'm on and everything else. I've been on psychiatric drugs for so long, the psychiatrist has written me off and everything else." I said: "What a load of crap!" I said: "You go out and ask a hundred people out there and I bet they're on something to keep them going for the day." I said: "If that's the way you feel, what's the point? You're feeling sorry for yourself, that you're having to take them (drugs) to keep you going through the day." I think I floored him. His reaction was he just 'sat' there. He said: "You're humouring me." I said: "I've never humoured you." I said: "We've always called a spade a spade." He wouldn't actually say "Yes, or no." Then afterwards he turned around and said: "Well, I've got a bit more living to do" and I said: "Good, I'm glad," so I gave him another hug.'

Relating to one another's humanness. Max knew Jane as a person with a family. Jane said:

> 'He knows a fair bit about me. I have talked a lot about my family and that, because this morning when I was so rapt with Leonie [Jane's daughter] getting the uni place, he said: "Hang about , she's only about three foot high," and I said: "No, she's 18!" and he said: "Oh, yeah, that's right."

Max also assisted Jane with some of her postregistration study.

> 'I was doing philosophy last year and he'd also studied philosophy. So I brought my books in and said: 'Here you are. You can write my first essay for me.' [Max was] probably not [helpful] in the sense of really knowing much about Descartes or Hume or whatever, but he appeared interested. He allowed me to sort of spout off a bit.'

Jane knew Max as a person, who was worth the time she spent with him in straight talk and encouragement. She said:

> 'I don't know, he's never actually turned around and said to me, like I've said to him, "I like you. You're a nice guy." He's never actually turned around and said, "Hey, you're a nice person" either, but from the vibes I get, I think that that's what he's thinking. I hope he's thinking that anyway. I think he is a person that is very guarded with his emotions and he puts himself down a heck of a lot...He's a nice guy, he puts himself down just too much, he's an intelligent guy. I can see the frustration in him. He's been encapsulated in this body that just won't do things for him, he's really quite frustrated. I like him as a person.'

Expressing feelings. After the straight talking session between them both, Max cried and Jane explained how she was feeling.

> 'I felt good, because I was crying as well. The eye contact wasn't there first of all, but when he said: "I've got some living to do," he looked straight at me and I felt "Oh!" I said: "Wasn't this the real Max that we saw the first time?" He said: "No, you wouldn't like the real Max." And I said: "Why?" He said: "Because I'd be in the looney bin" and I said: "Well you'd be in good company then wouldn't you." He looked at me. I said: "We'd all be over there with you," I said, "Because we all hide a certain amount of ourselves and we just put over what we want to put over to people." Since then he's been laughing and joking and the snide remarks are back again. Even the girl [nurse] on nights the following morning said: "I just can't get over the improvement in him." I said: "I don't know, he could have been ready to say [to himself] you know get a hold of yourself." But I said: "No, I'm going to give myself a pat on the back. I deserve it". He's a nice guy.'

Jane expressed how she felt in relation to being the one to discuss with Max whether or not he wished to be resuscitated, should his heart stop beating.

'I don't know. I've said basically a lot of my nursing is gut feeling. I can't explain, but I think I'll know [when the time comes to discuss resuscitation with Max]...I think it will feel bloody awful. I'm not looking forward to it one little bit...Personally, myself I would like that choice [of whether or not I wanted to be resuscitated]...But I'm just thinking of Max as a person, as a patient being poked at or whatever you want to put a label on it. I just think that he has that right [to decide for himself].'

Jane expressed her feelings about herself as a person and a professional.

'I think what you see is what you get. I take a lot of my work home, I must admit. I worry a lot about them [the patients] and I find it hard to turn off...I think I'm crazy sometimes. I think that's why I enjoy being in here [the PNU], because it gives you a chance to be yourself, to get closer to the patients. [In an intensive care situation] you're too concerned about the tubes, the bags and the bits and pieces to think that there is actually a person in that bed, that needs to be taken care of. My eyes fill, and this is me, I feel sometimes "God you're an idiot." But I just can't help it, the eyes fill up and I think "Gee, I should be harder." But I can't even begin to put a defence mechanism, I wouldn't know where to start, because that wouldn't be me. Should I become more immune? That wouldn't be me. I might just as well go out of nursing then.'

Conclusions

Max was alone, battling out each day in his head, feeling there was no point to it all, but holding on to what he had. He had down days and of late he had been very depressed. He had demonstrated this with outbursts of anger at the nursing staff. Jane and Max knew each other as nurse and patient over the two occasions in which Max had been admitted to the PNU. They had developed a rapport, which Jane described as 'calling a spade a spade.'

Jane came back after being on holidays and was surprised to see that Max had altered from how she remembered him. He answered with resignation her offer to help move him for pressure care and she challenged him. Jane knew Max and she would not let him retreat into self pity. She challenged him to stop feeling sorry for himself. He told her that he had not been able to show anyone who he really was, for fear that he would be put into the 'looney bin.' He called a spade a spade and so did she, so he had met his match in Jane. She would not let him wallow in self-pity and she let him know that how he was feeling mattered to her. Their straight talking together helped to stir him out of his despondency.

The focus of their interaction was a very intimate procedure, which had its amusing side. The regular bowel evacuation procedure, which Jane and Max undertook together, was a well known event amongst the nursing staff on the unit. It had been symbolised in the form of a joke amongst the nursing staff; a chocolate box containing a piece of fake faeces, which was presented to Jane at a staff party.

Jane decided to share the joke with Max and presented the box to him the next time the bowel evacuation procedure was due to be done. He knew the presentation was coming; it was a 'set up job,' but he went along with it, because it was fun and he knew that Jane knew how he would react. They humoured each other, yet they also respected each other. In the everyday world, it takes a lot of understanding between friends before you can joke about something as personal as bowel habits.

The bowel evacuation was an everyday procedure for them both. Max explained it as something that had to be done, which they both knew how to manage, so it was not an embarrassment to either of them. They continued to talk together throughout the procedure about the possible causes of the emptiness of Max's bowel. The outside world of the unit went on as usual, while, behind the screens, Jane worked with Max on the evacuation of his bowel. Later, Jane and Max talked about family and friends as she washed Max's genitals with total absorption and care. This was their usual world; being together during intimate procedures, which had to be done, but were done, nevertheless, with artistic sensitivity and skill.

Jane thought of Max as a nice person, who was intelligent. She felt that he was trapped in his paralysed body and she cared about how that might feel for him. As well as being there for him with her nursing knowledge and skills, Jane shared her personal self with Max. Max knew a lot about Jane's family, her studies, and her way of talking straight with him when she thought he needed it. In return, he was 'straight' with her. Theirs was a special relationship built on mutual respect for their shared humanity. Something as intimate as a bowel evacuation was simultaneously serious and humorous, because they understood one another and they were aware of how far they could go before offending one another's sensitivities.

Introducing Vicky

Vicky was born on 1 June 1910. She lives with her daughter and involves herself fully in the domestic duties. Vicky has insulin-

dependent diabetes mellitus and she has beèn admitted to the PNU
to assist her in stabilising her blood sugar levels. In the last few
days, Vicky has noticed some numbness in her left hand.

Jane and Vicky: a story about days when everything seems to go wrong

Vicky is sitting on her bed, looking sad and tearful. I listen to her
while she tells me about her left hand, how 'it is no good,' and how
she might as well die. She looks up and says: 'God, take me now!'
She tells me about all the housework she does and shows me the
crocheting she is doing. She says that she doesn't want to become
useless. Drips fall from her nose. She catches some with her
crumpled tissue paper. She is a picture of utter despondency.

Later, I see her in the shower. Jane is helping her to dry herself
and get dressed. She has her head down and she is weeping in
between comments to Jane. Jane is asking her whether she
understands about her diet. 'You were eating a banana this
morning,' she says. 'Not good?' Vicky asks in her lyrical Italian
accent. 'No, not really. I've asked the dietitian to come to have a
talk with you,' says Jane. 'Are oranges alright?' Vicky asks. 'Yes,
but they must be eaten at certain times.' 'I won't eat, if I not
allowed,' she says dejectedly, 'I not hungry.'

They both continue with drying Vicky's body. She is a thin
woman, of fairly short stature. Around her neck she wears her
religious medals. Jane asks her to stand up so they can dry the
remaining parts of her body and she stands inside her walking
frame. Jane asks whether she can dry her bottom. She says she
cannot, because her hand is too sore. Jane dries her bottom and
hands her the talcum powder. Vicky shakes some of the powder
into her right hand and pats it on her chest. Further attempts
meet with the talc container falling to the shower floor. On the
third and last occasion, Vicky looks upwards and implores God to
take her. 'I can't eat what I want to! I can't do what I want to!
What life is this?' she asks.

Jane speaks soothingly to her and tells her that it mightn't be all
that bad and assures her that we all have days in which everything
seems to be going wrong. Jane slows down her movements and
continues to talk reassuringly and Vicky settles down. Jane asks
her to sit down, so she can put her pants on and Vicky says it's wet.
Jane tells her she has put a towel down on the shower chair, so
Vicky sits down.

Jane hands the petticoat to Vicky. It is inside out and Vicky cannot sort out which way to put it on, so Jane lets her try for a while and then helps her to orient the garment. Vicky puts on her dress and Jane kneels down on the shower room floor to put Vicky's pants on. As she stands, Jane pulls them into position. Vicky's posture is looking slumped and tired.

As they are about to move from the shower area, a 'polished' voice is heard across the partition. 'I'm going to the toilet next door here,' Ruth announces. 'That's OK,' replies Jane. 'It's just that I have to open the door next to you and you may not see it,' says Ruth. 'Oh, I see. Thank you,' responds Jane.

Vicky is shuffling forward in the frame. The shower curtain is pulled back and time is allowed for Ruth to go into the toilet and close her door. Vicky goes to the basin and at Jane's suggestion, washes her teeth in some water. Andrew walks into the area and asks where Ruth is. We indicate the toilet door. He walks into the shower area and calls over the toilet wall that Ruth won't be able to go home today as anticipated, because there are workers in her driveway. She asks for further clarification and it feels like there is a lot of noise and people in a small space.

At the basin, Vicky gives a shudder and starts to cry. Jane notices and walks in beside her to comfort her. They move off together and Sue comes to the door and asks Jane about a drug entry. She sees me in the shower room also and says: 'Oh, you're doing an interaction.' Jane gives Sue an explanation related to the drug entry and Sue goes off down the corridor.

Jane hands me Vicky's hand basin containing her toiletries and I walk behind them down the corridor. Vicky is still upset about her hand and what it might mean to her life. Jane is talking with her, telling her the doctor is coming to see her later and encouraging her to take care with her walking. There is movement in the corridor. A theatre trolley is near the door. People are moving near the nurses' desk. We go into the room and the theatre trolley follows soon after us; it is for the woman in the bed opposite. She is standing in a pink hospital gown and the attendant asks her how she is. 'Do you really want to know?' she asks. He doesn't reply as he helps her onto the trolley.

Jane is helping to put Vicky's things away in her locker. Vicky is sitting on the end of the bed. Jane locates her comb and Vicky combs her hair. Opposite us, Sue is giving her opinions of men as a general group. Something has happened recently. She apologises to the woman on the trolley for not having her ready for the

Operating Theatre. 'They surprised us,' she says. 'Another man!' she says, looking at the theatre attendant. He smiles and looks at us and says to himself: 'I will not respond to that. It might alarm them.' They leave and Andrew walks in and tidies the woman's bed and talks to Jane about Ruth's husband. 'He is not ready for her to come home. The drive is full of workers. That's fair enough. But no food in the house. That's not right!'

By now, Vicky is walking with Jane to the table in the centre of the room. They discuss where she will sit and she settles in the chair. The tears have stopped and the room is quiet.

Interpretations

Vicky was an Italian woman, who could speak English as a second language, but not well enough to understand the nuances of her diabetes management. Jane attempted to explain to Vicky that she needed to be careful about her diet in relation to her insulin dosage, but Vicky misunderstood, thinking that it was yet another deprivation in her already austere existence. Vicky was most concerned about some changes she had noticed in her hand. On this occasion of nursing care, Jane had been assisting Vicky to shower and dress herself and the day seemed to be going along quite forlornly for them both.

I analysed the text relating to the interaction between Jane and Vicky and five main qualities and activities emerged, which were: appreciating help; expressing feelings; calming fears; recognising the days in which everything seems to go wrong; and being part of the everyday life of the unit. These qualities and activities will be discussed in the section that follows.

Appreciating help. Vicky was appreciative of the help Jane and the other nurses gave her. She said:

> 'Good. Help me, put me the water, just no hot no cold and give me the towel, the soap, I wash myself and then rinse me and then make me dry, really really good. Very good…I can't go to the toilet, give me the pan and to help me…It's good…Help. Help, quickly help…I can. I manage (to help myself)…They help me, help me.'

Expressing feelings. Vicky had a tearful morning, but it soon abated. She said she was feeling upset.

> 'Oh, about my hand, yes, upset and I cry. Come in the nurse, she say it going to be alright.'

Jane knew that Vicky was upset and so she helped her finish dressing so that she could get back to her room. Jane explained:

'You have to stand back, but I ended up putting her slip on, because
although she's got it sort of in between her teeth and trying to do
it—"There's no way," I thought, "Even if I just pop it over her
head, at least she's got a start." I think I just automatically put her
dress on for her, because I just thought "It's just getting too
distressing for her. I'm just going to finish it as quick as I can and
get her back to her room."'

Calming fears. Vicky was upset and worried during her shower.
She did not understand her diabetic diet and she was extremely
agitated about the lack of power in her hand. Jane kept reassuring
Vicky that the dietitian would help with her diet and that the doctor
would visit to look at her hand. I told Vicki that I noticed that she was
trying to put some powder on herself and that she dropped the
container a few times. I asked her how that made her feel. Vicki replied:

*'Ah yes. They give it to me again and they say: "Don't worry, don't
worry."'*

Recognising the days in which everything seems to go wrong.
Jane reassured Vicky that on some days everything seems to go wrong.
    I wrote these notes in my journal:

'Jane speaks soothingly to her (Vicky) and tells her that it
mightn't be all that bad and assures her that we all have days in
which everything seems to be going wrong. Jane slows down her
movements and continues to talk reassuringly and Vicky settles
down. Jane asks her to sit down so she can put her pants on and
Vicky says it's wet. Jane tells her she has put a towel down on the
shower chair, so Vicky sits down.'

Jane felt that it was true for her that on 'some days everything
seems to go wrong.' She said:

'And everything has gone wrong since!...Well I started off really
quite well, I thought, "Gee we're doing really well" and it ended
up a real shit of a day (excuse my French!)'.

Jane related a story, that unfolded that same day, of an interaction
with a doctor. He threatened to transfer Vicky to another ward,
because she had some neurological deficit in her hand, which he
thought had not been reported. Jane had reported it to the Resident
Medical Officer, but the message had not been passed on to the
Honorary Medical Officer. What resulted was an incident which made
Jane feel fairly incompetent and frustrated. She concluded that on
some days she felt more able to speak up than others and that she had
acted as well as she could have, given the circumstances. She explained:

'I do that [find voice]. There are some days that I can just come out with things just like that and then other days...I just stood there and I thought, "Well if you want to move her, move her." But it leaves a bad taste in your mouth. I suppose you start to question yourself a bit to say: "Well. I'm only human. I only did what I thought was right."'

Being part of the everyday life of the unit. There was a general sense of busyness and clamour in the unit that day.

I wrote some notes about the context in my journal, describing the clamour of the shared space in the shower area and the ward. The context was a very public world, in which a lot was happening at one time, unselfconsciously. The clamour and the busyness of that day seemed to me to be like the way a noisy family group might rattle around together inside their home if it was raining outside, and they could not get out temporarily.

Conclusions

Vicky was miserable with pain and feelings of change in her right hand. She was anxious about what it might mean to her lifestyle, because she worked hard and she enjoyed craftwork. She was a picture of despondency, immersed fully in her experience of anxiety and hopelessness.

She had a shower assisted by Jane, and she remained fairly despondent throughout, wailing periodically for God's deliverance. Vicky's concern about her hand and her confusion about her diabetic diet seemed to give her scant room for much joy in her world that day. Jane usually allowed Vicky to do as much as possible for herself, but on this particular day, Vicky's efforts to help herself were impeded by the loss of power in her hand, so Jane assisted her as much as possible. Jane tried to console Vicky by saying that the doctor had been told about her concern and that he was coming to look at her hand. Jane attempted to discuss Vicky's diabetic diet with her, but it created more of a sense of hopelessness in Vicky, who misunderstood the notion of diabetic exchanges and interpreted Jane's words as evidence of further limitations to her independence.

Jane continued to console her and to make her comfortable. Vicky began to settle down after she was back in bed and her daughter was with her. The unit was humming with busyness that day. The motion of ward life was evident around Vicky and Jane; they weaved their way in and around it as they continued their interaction. It was a day which seemed fairly joyless for the both of them. Vicky was caught up in her despair and Jane became embroiled in a conflict of her own.

Weaved into Jane and Vicky's interaction that day, there was some confusion over the reporting function of the nurses in the unit. Jane expressed a gamut of emotions, when she related how Vicky's doctor threatened to transfer Vicky out of the unit. All in all, Jane and Vicky had both had a terrible day. Regardless of their personal plights, the clamour of the day in the unit continued around them. The unselfconscious dialogue between nurses and patients in the bathroom and back in Vicky's room, attested to their sense of familiarity in the context.

All the people interacted in their respective 'bubbles of reality,' bumping against and merging into one another's realities, as the flow of their Being-in-the-world of the unit unfolded that day. It was as though the sum total of people's experiences saturated the ambience of the unit. Jane recognised that some days are not so easy to live through as others. The next day, Vicky was walking on her frame and her wailing had ceased. Jane also felt reconstituted and coped with whatever her day brought forth. It seems that in day to day life we experience highs and lows; this is in tune with the polar nature of our existence as human beings.

6. Peter's nurse-patient interactions

Introducing Peter

Peter began his nurse training in 1976. He had no intention of being a nurse and worked in a bank for two years and 'absolutely despised it.' His mother is a nurse and she suggested that he apply to do nursing, and the more he thought about it, the more he thought it was a good idea. For Peter, nursing is about helping people to help themselves, and he believes that his role is to teach people, so they can do things to be as independent as is possible for them. Peter finds nursing is very challenging and stimulating intellectually, because it makes him learn about other people and about himself. Peter thinks that 'nursing units and the switch to tertiary nursing are good' and he hopes they will help people to see what nurses are doing and why they are doing it. He is concerned about the tendency in Australia to treat health care as a business, so that elective surgery gets more attention than other areas, such as the care of the elderly, and mental health.

Introducing Jean

Jean was born on 15 April 1929. She lives at home with her husband and they have a happy family life with their grown children and their grandchildren. Jean developed insulin dependent diabetes after ten years on oral hypoglycaemics and she is in the PNU to learn how to manage her insulin replacement.

Peter and Jean: a story about patient education

Peter says that they are ready when I am, so I save the information on the computer and go into the sitting room opposite, where Jean and Peter are seated at the end of the table. Jean is an alert looking, bright-faced woman, dressed in a summer frock. She is talking with Peter about what she comprehends of diabetes thus far. Yesterday she saw some videos and Peter tells her he wants to see how much she understood.

He begins by asking her what she thinks diabetes is. She answers that it is to do with sugar and says that it becomes high. He nods and continues on from what she has said, by talking about insulin and the pancreas. She knows the word 'pancreas' and points to the area on her abdomen in which it situated. He tells her about glucose and cells and how insulin works to help the transport of sugar from the bloodstream to body cells. She listens intently and asks questions and seeks confirmation for things about which she is unclear.

They talk together for at least ten minutes about the effects and management of diabetes. She says there is so much to know and she admits that she never really took it seriously before. She says she will be more alert now. He says her friends at the bowling club should know she is a diabetic. She says they know already and that they keep an eye on her. She said she didn't realise that she should carry barley sugar, but it will be the first thing she buys when she gets out of hospital.

Peter checks that she understands why the barley sugar may be needed and what to do, should she have a hypoglycaemic reaction. He says he also feels her husband should know more, but she is opposed firmly to that just yet, because he is getting ready to have another operation and she doesn't want to worry him about herself.

Peter suggests she view the video on foot care and sick days. He gives her the reading that accompanies the video and tells her that she should only concentrate on that. They talk about discharge plans. She would like to go home for her granddaughter's christening on Sunday, so Peter projects Saturday as the discharge day. He explains the education program will be completed, but that it will depend on how well her blood sugar is stabilised by the insulin. She understands, but she says that she would prefer to get out on Friday if that is possible, because a daughter is arriving from Queensland. Peter writes ('possibly Friday') because he won't be working on Friday and it will make it apparent to the other nurses that that is what Jean would prefer, if it is possible.

They seem to complete their talk, so I thank them both and leave after arranging to talk with them separately later. I go to my office across the passageway and I hear their voices about ten minutes later. They are still talking. I think that there is so much to talk about. Laughter comes across the hallway from time to time. I think how precious it must be to have time to talk and be listened to, when you need to understand something upon which your health depends.

Interpretations

When I used the method of analysis I described in Chapter 2, I found six main qualities and activities emerged from the text relating to the interaction between Peter and Jean, which appeared to illuminate the phenomenon of ordinariness in nursing. They were: appreciating skilful nursing care; acknowledging one another's humanness; approving commendable human qualities; acknowledging specialness in everyday situations; acknowledging the importance of family and home; and appreciating a 'home-like' atmosphere.

Appreciating skilful nursing care. Jean appreciated the way in which Peter taught her what she felt she needed to know. She said:

> 'Well, I feel that he [Peter] explains things very plain to you, I mean, more than any one I've been to thus far. The people where I've been use big words and I don't understand, but he puts it in English that I can understand. That's what I like about being here [in the unit] at the moment. I went up from that talk yesterday and picked up the papers and it made sense to me. When the doctors talk, they talk in big words that don't make any sense. Peter breaks it down into words [I can understand], that's what I like, ever since I've been here. That's why I like him.'

Peter took his role of diabetes educator seriously and acknowledged patients' responsibilities in their own care. He explained:

> 'I think it [the role of diabetes educator] is very important, because if we can get people to look after their own care, be responsible for their own care, they are going to have a lot less problems in later life. They are at risk of heart attack, eyes problems, having a leg off. It's best to get onto it [diabetes management] now, not ten years on down the track. I don't think you can just say: "Right, this is what you have got to learn!" You've got to impress on them that it's their responsibility really. I tell them I can teach them so much and once they leave here, it is up to them. They are responsible for looking after themselves.'

Acknowledging one another's humanness. Jean understood her own learning capabilities.

> 'That [the rate of learning] is good! I can only do so far. Maybe some people have got a quicker brain than me, but I haven't felt well for a few months. I think that's what it is. It is taking me a little bit longer to grasp what he is saying, but I've got to get away on my own and do it. That's the only way I've been able to do something I wanted to do. I let it sink in by studying quietly…I've made up my mind to buy this set of books, so when I feel I don't understand something that is happening to me, I'm going to read it and try to work out what it is…I'm not dumb, but, as I said, I just felt it was mumbo-jumbo. I feel that I can cope with it since yesterday and I jot things down on paper so that I feel that I

understand it...Last night I sat down and studied by writing it down in
my own words. I'm going to study it my own way and then I'll make up
my mind whether I've got it exactly.'

Peter realised that his teaching processes would need to be tailored
to Jean's needs. He explained:

'Well, someone like Jean—it needs to be very simple and specific.
You can't have very technical terms, because it wouldn't mean a
thing to her. But younger adults, who are used to that sort of
language, well you can actually be a bit more technical. With others,
you have to do it in layman's terms...Jean is very keen to learn, but
she finds that too much information at any one particular time
tends to overload her and she tends to get a bit confused about
things, so you have to be careful not to go too far ahead too quickly.'

Peter also acknowledged his own human tendency to want to move
forward too rapidly.

'Especially me, I get a bit too keen [laugh] and [tend to want to do
too much].'

Approving commendable human qualities. Jean and Peter
approved of some commendable qualities they recognised in each
other. Jean said:

'Peter is excellent. I think he is good.'

And Peter said:

'I think she is very cheerful.'

Acknowledging specialness in everyday situations. Even
though diabetes education was a part of Peter's everyday work role,
Jean felt that he had done it especially for her.

'It was special, because I thought he was doing it for me, you know,
that's how I felt...To be honest, I hadn't even thought of anybody else.
I thought he was doing that especially for me...At first he gave me a
whole heap of these books and then he took them off me and said: 'No, I
think two at a time is enough.' He saw that I was struggling to understand
it...I felt as though it was just for me. I hope he can keep getting through
to people like he got through to me.'

Acknowledging the importance of family and home. Jean was
immersed in her family life and she was trying to learn as much as
she could about managing her diabetes, so that she could go home
to be with them all again. Jean knew that her family would help her
to keep learning and living with her diabetes.

'I'll get my kids to query me on it when I get home, because I've got
children who will help me. I think it's the only way when you've got this

[diabetes mellitus]. I've had enough sickness in my life. I want to get on top of this. I've had cancer and I've had a heart attack, so I'm not going to give in to this. I'm going to beat it if I can, or live with it anyway.'

Jean wanted to go home and she acknowledged the help of a nurse in conquering her fear of giving herself her insulin needle.

'Well, with the needle, until this morning, I was frightened. I live next to a woman, who has the nursing sister come in every day to have the needle. She just can't do it for herself. But, I know now that I could do it. I could help her after even just this one thing this morning. I was really frightened, but the nurse, whoever she was, was wonderful. She said: "Do this, do this..." and I did it before I thought about it. No, I won't be frightened going home now.'

That week promised to be particularly eventful for Jean and her family. She was thinking especially of her eldest grand-daughter, with whom she had a special bond.

'This week, a lot [is happening]! I just wish I could be on top of it. Everything's happening. My granddaughter is having a baby within the next hour, a granddaughter is getting christened on Sunday. We are a very close family, you've got to understand this. I've got two daughters past forty and one who is twenty-seven. There are four girls and two boy grandchildren. They are all coming together this weekend. You can imagine what it is going to be like. The grandparents of the one who is to be christened are Italian and they are so wonderful. Can you imagine what it will be like? It was going to be a small celebration, but with Italians, it never is. I tell myself not to get upset; I try not to, but this is my eldest granddaughter, who is having the baby. She is a girl who comes in to see me on her way to work, and has breakfast with me. You can see she is special. She said to me: "Nan, you'll come to hospital with me?" This was last week. I sat with her for two days. I took her for walks and that. I said: "I'll be there, lovie." I didn't expect to come into hospital myself! She'll be right. She has her own mother with her. I'd like to have been there, I really would have. Oh, yes, she knows that. She knows I'll be there. When she sees me, she's going to put her arms around me and cry. When she gets excited or—can you imagine what it is going to be like?'

Peter was aware of Jean's absorption in her family.

'She will also become a great grandmother today, so...Yes, I just had a phone call now, saying it [the baby] is on the way.'

Appreciating a 'home-like' atmosphere. Jean appreciated the atmosphere in the PNU.

'Well, the nursing here, to me, is wonderful. I think this sort of thing is wonderful. You can have your visitors. You are in your own clothes. You don't feel like it is a hospital. You feel like they (the nurses) are right there! I feel it is a different thing. Like they (the nurses) are...you don't feel embarrassed or anything. I've been in and out of hospital and

they are no different to other nurses as far as skill goes, but they are different, something is there, I feel, but I can't put my finger on it yet. There is no uniform. I wonder whether it is that? When I was walking past a nursing sister I used to stop and think... They have taken away the authority here. That's it! That's what I feel it is!'

Conclusions

Jean loved her family and was longing to go home to be with them. She had been through a lot of illness herself and she regarded the need for insulin to treat her diabetes as something else she could learn to live with. She had not really taken her diabetes seriously till the time in which she found herself in the PNU. There was too much else to do rather than to make a fuss about her own condition.

She had survived cancer and was continuing to help her husband through his illness, so her diabetes had not impacted on her as something of which she should be especially conscious. Her husband had been ill and was due to go into hospital, so she did not want him to know that she needed insulin. His state of mind was more important to her than her need to tell him about her insulin-dependent diabetes. She was willing to be open with her family and her bowling club friends about her diabetes, but she wanted to shield her husband from this latest development for a while.

She tried to apply herself to learning and she knew that it took a lot for things to sink in with her, so she tried extra hard to retain what Peter told her. Peter taught Jean at the rate she could manage. He knew he needed to take it 'slowly and surely,' for Jean to gain the best benefit from the educational sessions. She liked Peter's teaching style, because he put concepts into words she understood and he took things at a pace to suit her. She was trying as hard as she could, so that she could return to her family and cope as well as she could. Jean's was a big, happy, energetic family and she wanted to be as active in it as soon as possible.

Peter knew she was expecting to hear news of her granddaughter on that day, the one to whom Jean was especially close. Her granddaughter's baby was due any minute and Peter understood Jean's excitement and apprehension; he was sharing it with her.

Jean was more to Peter than just someone who had diabetes; she was a person with family ties and a personality of her own. He was trying to get Jean out of the unit in time for the weekend, so that she could be part of the family celebrations. The education sessions were almost finished and it was more a matter of getting Jean stabilised on insulin, so that she was ready to go home.

The teaching sessions between Jean and Peter were often for relatively large chunks of time, and Peter had to take into consideration the other patients' needs for nursing care, with whom he dealt simultaneously. There was so much to talk about. Peter made time to talk with Jean and to listen to her. She needed to understand so much, upon which her future health and happiness depended.

Introducing Vernon

Vernon was born on 3 May 1902. He had been living at home with his daughter in accommodation in her back yard; however, Vernon was most recently in a nursing home for respite care, because his daughter felt that she could not care for him on her own. Vernon was admitted to the PNU from the nursing home, where he had a fall. He is having episodes of pulselessness, followed by nausea, sometimes accompanied by vomiting and several days of fatigue. He does not want to be resuscitated. His only wish is that he will not die in pain.

Peter and Vernon: a story about facing death with humour

The buzzer sounds from the men's toilet, so Peter goes to retrieve Vernon and I meet them both as they are entering the shower room. I greet Vernon and we all go into the shower room and shut the door. The room is small and warm. There is a residual odour of faeces coming from the toilet next door. Peter is preparing himself by putting on his plastic apron. He already has plastic covering over his shoes.

Vernon is standing next to the shower chair. He is a tall, thin man. He is dressed in his pyjamas. Peter assists him to sit down on the shower chair. He lets himself down carefully, searching for the arm of the plastic chair to guide himself down. Vernon's head is round. He has a bald surface on the top of his head and his grey hair, eyebrows and growing beard, suggest a man of advanced years. His movements are careful and tentative. His long fingers start to undo the buttons on his pyjamas top, while Peter tries to undo the knot on Vernon's pyjamas pants.

Peter tells him that the knot will not untie easily, so Vernon lifts himself slightly on the chair so that Peter can pull the pants off still tied. He sits there with knee pads on, which he tells me have magnets in them to help his arthritis. When I ask him whether they are of any use, he claims they are effective. Vernon makes small noises with each exertion, but he moves himself whenever he is requested to, or whenever he chooses.

The pyjamas are off and Vernon is sitting naked in the small, warm shower room. Peter adjusts the water and begins to wet Vernon's body. Peter hands a face cloth to Vernon and tells him what it is. Peter quietly tells me aside that Vernon is seventy percent blind. I connect Peter's explanation of Vernon's partial blindness to the explanation of the cloth and soap approaching. Vernon begins to soap the cloth and wash his face. He begins to puff quietly. He tells Peter that he feels breathless. Peter offers to help and Vernon takes up the offer. Peter asks Vernon whether it is OK to tell me a bit about him.

Vernon agrees readily and Peter tells me that Vernon has been living with his daughter. 'Not living with her,' Vernon butts in, 'I had a bungalow in her back yard.' 'He is 89, will be 90 soon...' More conversation ensues, mainly between Peter and Vernon, in order to get the details clear, by making sure that Vernon agrees with what Peter is saying. They talk easily together. Peter seems to know a lot about Vernon, not only in relation to this present condition, but also in relation to who and how Vernon is as a person.

'Unfortunately, he took a fall, so he is in here to get mobile again,' Peter explains. 'Maybe you could show Bev your photos of your eighty-ninth birthday!' suggests Peter. 'Oh, Peter!' replies Vernon in lighthearted exasperation. They both smile. 'Who hasn't seen them!' Vernon looks over to me and talks to me as Peter continues to wash his body. 'I showed them to a doctor and he said he would have liked to have been there with his video recorder.' 'It sounds like it was a great time,' I say.

The lighthearted chatter goes on fairly continuously. It is about how good Vernon is for his age, his impending birthday, and the nature of Vernon's 'funny turns' he has been having. Peter continues to wash and shower Vernon's body throughout the conversation. He suggests that Vernon may like to wash his own 'privates,' and hands the cloth to Vernon, who does so with great thoroughness. There seems to be little or no self-consciousness here. Peter offers to wash Vernon's hair. As he is lathering the soap into his hair, Peter comments on Vernon's lack of hair. A few brief words are exchanged and then Vernon looks at Peter and says: 'You have a small head.' By this time Peter is wiping elsewhere and quips: 'Thank you very much Vernon. I love you too!' They both laugh.

It is time to complete the shower. Peter turns off the taps and gives a towel to Vernon. He wipes the parts he can reach easily and Peter wipes the other parts, which are relatively difficult to reach, such as Vernon's legs, toes and back. Vernon then wipes his groin and we help him to stand upright, while Peter wipes his buttocks. The conversation continues throughout the drying process. The activity is at Vernon's pace; if he is puffing audibly, Peter slows the activity down.

Vernon sits on the dry towel placed under his buttocks on the chair and Peter hands him his clean shirt in a way which would mean that it would need to be passed around Vernon's back to be put on. Vernon intervenes and takes the shirt telling Peter that that is not the way he does it. He adjusts the shirt so that he can put both hands through the top and pass it over his back to then pull down. He explains that this way means he doesn't have to search around the back for the other sleeve. Peter is happy with that. He stands back and lets Vernon do it his way.

Vernon remains seated while Peter puts the underpants, pants, socks and slippers on the lower end of Vernon's body. Each garment rests on the dry towel under Vernon's feet until Vernon stands up and the pants are taken the rest of the way up his body in one movement. Vernon decides that he may need a peri-pad (pad between the legs), when Peter reminds him that these are his last pair of clean trousers. We position a large, wide incontinence pad between Vernon's legs. I wonder how he feels about wearing one of these things. 'Let's see you do up this belt!' jests Vernon, as Peter brings the belt around the front to secure it. Peter meets the challenge and fastens the buckle. The trousers pucker on the belt and the belt pulls well around Vernon's thin waist. 'We'll need the walking frame,' says Peter, so I take that as my cue to get it from outside the outer door. Vernon takes it and moves off slowly.

Peter tells Vernon he'll take him into the room next to his own for a while, because work people are in Vernon's room putting in wiring for air-conditioning. We go into the room and Vernon lets himself down into a chair. Peter makes sure Vernon is comfortable and I clean up the shower-room. Vernon has had his shower for today.

Interpretations

Vernon was 89 years old, and of late he was subject to sudden pulselessness and collapse. He was aware that his life was ending and his only wish was that it would be a painless passing. He remembered his last birthday, and the stripper, who had performed then had been a subject of conversation ever since. Vernon enjoyed a sense of fun and he appreciated nurses sharing a joke with him. Vernon respected Peter, because Peter motivated him to help himself as much as possible, yet he was gentle and kind to him. The nurse-patient interaction in this case evolved around a shower time, in which Peter assisted Vernon to cleanse and dress himself.

I analysed the text relating to the interaction between Peter and Vernon and eight main qualities and activities emerged, which were: enjoying a sense of humour; approving commendable human qualities; talking straight; equating with a sense of 'that's all'; relating to one another's humanness; balancing helping and not helping ; acknowledging specialness in everyday situations; and expressing feelings.

Enjoying a sense of humour. Vernon had a sense of humour, which seemed to lighten his circumstances. Peter said of him:

> 'I think he's [Vernon is] a great old man. He's got a good sense of humour. A bit frisky sometimes, gets a bit frisky with the girls, some of them...Yeah he gets a bit cheeky...He's got a bit of spunk and a bit of life in him. It is unfortunate that his daughter doesn't feel that she can look after him any more.'

Vernon shared his humour freely, evidenced in his quips with Peter during the shower and in his enjoyment in relating the story about the stripper.

Approving commendable human qualities. Vernon approved of Peter's gentleness, a quality which he compared to other nurses. Vernon said:

> *'He's a good man, a helluva good man. I've got no gripes, I'm quite happy with him...He's a very gentle man, Peter. He knows every move you should make and he makes you do it, that's what I like about him...It's his nature...Peter is a gentle man. Peter doesn't hurry you. He just says: "Say when you're ready. Sing out." Nice lad that one.'*

Talking straight. Vernon and Peter were both men, who spoke clearly about what they thought. Vernon gave Peter the right to speak his mind, just as he gave it to himself. Vernon explained:

> *'I didn't like it [having to get out of bed], I had to get out of bed! No, he [Peter] just gives the orders and they all just spring to attention...There's no mucking about with Peter. He calls a spade a spade and I like it. If I've got anything to say, I'll damn well say it, whether it slips out or not, it comes out...Yes. Quite happy with Peter.'*

Equating with a sense of 'that's all'. Vernon managed his world
to some extent, by experiencing it as something which had to be
tolerated as being reasonable and necessary. In relation to how he
dealt with being washed by other people, he used his sense of
humour, peppered with a sense of 'that's all there is to it!'

> *'Oh, not really [there's nothing different about Peter washing me]. You
> could rub me down anyway, the same as him I suppose. I sit in the chair
> and he does my knees and then he does my back and arms and my chest,
> but I wash the old personal and that's about all there is to it, dear.
> That's all. I can do that [wash my penis]. I don't want them mucking
> around with that. That's what I can't understand; how all these nurses
> [can bear to be] mucking around with bloody old men, old droopy grubs
> hangin' here there and everywhere...Don't affect me, love...Well, I've
> had nearly every nurse in [the town] wait on me. Back at my daughter's
> place the district nurses used to come out twice a week and shower me,
> but there was never anything spoken. I don't know, you've just got to
> put up with it I suppose...They [the district nurses] just treat it as a job
> and nothing else. A bit of love and care. They don't knock me around or
> anything. Everyday occurrence, love.'*

Relating to one another's humanness. Vernon realised that the
nurses were often busy and couldn't always attend to him instantly.
He said:

> *'I don't like it [having to wait for the buzzer to be answered]. They
> can't be everywhere at once. Some nights—it's just like the bell ringers
> here. It's ring, ring, ring everywhere, but I never trouble them of a night.
> I don't like to be an encumbrance on them.'*

Peter knew that Vernon's daughter was unable to manage her
father's care at her home, and that the aim of the nursing care was
to prepare Vernon for hostel placement, but Peter understood that,
within the reasonable dictates of humanness, it becomes necessary
to accept that some things can not be. Peter explained:

> 'He knows that [Vernon's daughter cannot manage looking after
> him]. But sometimes you've just got to accept that you can't do
> that any more and it's just become too much...He's not really up
> to hostel placement, but that's what we're trying to aim for him to
> do. We're trying to increase his mobility and things like that. They
> provide somebody to help him wash and things like that, so they'd
> be able to do that for him. But he needs to be able to walk fairly
> independently, which is where we're having the hard trouble
> actually. Some days he's better than others, but some days he's
> really poor with his mobility. So, he may have to end up in a nursing
> home.'

Balancing helping and not helping. Vernon was 89 years old,
and he was subject to collapse. Peter tried to find a balance between

what he would do for Vernon and what Vernon could do for himself. Peter assessed Vernon's capabilities constantly.

'Well, his walking's improved since yesterday. He wasn't walking very well at all yesterday. He seemed to be a lot more alert, a lot more chatty than he was yesterday. He was very tired and washed out. A general improvement. He needed to be directed to sit down onto the chair properly, as he always seems to forget, he tends tip backwards when he gets near a chair and reach out and grab things...He knows he's doing that [not sitting carefully], because when you tell him, he says: "Oh I forgot to do that" and he is quite humorous about it. He was able to help get himself undressed from top garments even though he had trouble with his pyjamas bottoms. The shower itself; he only made a halfhearted attempt at washing himself and, really, I had to end up doing it myself...Well, I thought because he's had these nasty fits, that perhaps maybe it had something to do with that. So I was a bit nervous at that stage [when Vernon was unable to wash himself], because he does become very sick at that point, but he seemed to settle down. I don't know whether it was some anxiety state or he just felt that he was doing too much.'

Peter acknowledged the difficulty in assessing Vernon's capabilities.

'Yes. It's difficult to know, because he's 89, nearly 90, and he's had a lot of help in the past. It's difficult to know how far to go to let him try and do it himself or to step in, and I sometimes wonder if I push him too hard, or I'm not asking him to do more for himself.'

Peter tried to explain how he assessed Vernon's capabilities on various occasions.

'It's difficult [to explain] really. It's his whole body language; the way he's trying to wash himself or not trying to wash himself. It's difficult to know, but when you look at him you just feel that he's not trying this and he doesn't particularly want to do that. I don't know what it is. It's difficult. I suppose that's what body language is all about, you just pick it up.'

In balancing Vernon's need for help, Peter differentiated between what he thought he could do for Vernon and what he might expect from someone else, who was not a nurse.

'She [Vernon's daughter] may be a bit too close. She'd feel like she needs to do more for him, instead of letting him do as much as he can, when he feels that he can manage for himself and so increases his independence. I think that is the thing, where we [nurses] have to actually know when to step in and when to stand back. I think that comes with training and experience. I don't think you can just pick up someone off the street and ask them to shower somebody and expect them to do it properly.'

Acknowledging specialness in everyday situations. Even though Vernon tended to describe his tolerance of having someone else shower him as something fairly inconsequential, Peter regarded the everyday routine of showering people, as a special time for being with patients. Peter said:

'I think it's quite important. For a start, they're undressed, and they are fully exposed to you, so therefore you have to actually get on well with them. It's very hard to give somebody a shower if they're feeling very self-conscious and things like that. So you've got to try and put them at their ease. With Vernon it's quite easy, because he's a jovial, jolly type of man anyway.'

Peter described the value of being with people during their daily shower, as quality time for talking together.

'Actually, I find it very easy to get a lot of information out of patients in the shower. They seem to be more willing to talk. I don't know if it's because they haven't got any clothes on...You couldn't get much more closer. They tell you a lot when they're in the shower. They tell you about their life and their expectations, what they're planning to do, and where they will be spending that day...For many of the patients, especially in the morning, it's probably the most time we spend with the patient, in the morning. We're very busy doing a lot of showers and a lot of washes. So you could spend up to half an hour, and that's a good long time. I don't know if they [patients] know that that's a good opportunity to tell the nurse what they do and things like that. But it's probably the most time we spend with a patient, in the morning particularly, when you can actually have quality time, when you've got their whole attention and they've got nothing else.'

Expressing feelings. Peter expressed some of the feelings he experienced in relation to giving nursing care, if he did not have time to be with patients.

'You get really frustrated when you've got loads and loads to do and you think how are you going to get it all done in the morning...Sometimes, if you feel a bit stressed out, you think: "I've got to rush rush rush," but you can't. You've got to stand back and let them [the patients] make their own mistakes.'

He expressed how he felt when Vernon corrected him about putting on his shirt after the shower.

'Obviously, I misinterpreted what he [Vernon] was trying to do. I thought he was trying to put his arm in the wrong sleeve. He wasn't. He knew exactly what he was going to do. He knew exactly how he was going to do it. I felt a fool then, because I felt that I'd gone too far (trying to help) that time. I should have let him carry on with what he was doing, because he knew what he was doing.'

Peter was surprised that Vernon was happy for me to be present in the shower room during their interaction. Peter compared Vernon's acceptance to how he might feel in the same situation.

'I was quite surprised at how well he took to somebody else being in there [the shower room] actually. I'm not sure if it had have been me in that position, whether I would like somebody else watching me. I was quite surprised about that.'

Conclusions

Vernon was an old man with a sense of humour and a love of fun. He had many showers assisted by nurses and he thought that it was an everyday occurrence, which didn't worry him. He mentioned that he tolerated it to some extent, and all he expected in return was some loving care and gentleness.

Vernon knew Peter called a spade a spade, and he liked that, because that was how he thought of himself. He became annoyed sometimes, when nurses made him wait, but he understood that they were busy and that some patients ring the bell often. So, Vernon was tolerant and allowed nurses the human qualities he allowed himself.

Peter encouraged him gently and joined in his fun. Vernon was happy to have Peter help him, because Peter was gentle and gave him encouragement. Vernon compared Peter to another nurse, who Vernon described as a 'bloody bull.' It seemed Vernon mainly required that nurses were gentle with him. The actual task of showering was inconsequential to Vernon, but he knew how he expected to be treated.

Vernon was not concerned unduly about having his genitals washed by someone else, although he preferred to do it himself to save someone else the task. Although he joked about his 'privates,' he described his alarm at nurses washing 'old, droopy grubs,' therefore, it seemed that he was reticent about sacrificing his privacy. Although Vernon made light of needing to be assisted in the shower, his messages were mixed about who might wash him, where and how.

Peter liked Vernon and he felt sorry that Vernon would not be able to go home to his daughter, but was destined to go to a nursing home. Peter wanted to make Vernon as independent as possible, so that he could have some choices about how and where he would end his days. Peter questioned himself constantly about the extent to which he could reasonably expect Vernon to be independent. He was aware of Vernon's age and his medical condition and he wanted to be as fair as possible to him. Peter assessed Vernon's capabilities daily to find a balance between helping him and allowing him to help himself. Peter seemed to know a lot about Vernon, not only in relation to this present condition, but also in relation to who and how Vernon was as a person.

In some ways, the shower was a challenge for them both. Vernon was exploring his physical limits and Peter was trying to allow him time and space to help himself. The potential of Vernon's sudden collapse was ever present, yet both men managed to keep a light approach to the showering. Vernon and Peter talked easily together. They exchanged comments in the shower about relative hair loss and head size and they laughed at the end of their banter. Peter respected Vernon and accepted his cheekiness. At 89 years of age, Vernon was quite a character in Peter's eyes.

Peter and Vernon went through this showering routine every second day, therefore, it was usual for the both of them. The day of the interaction was different, because I was present also. Peter was surprised at Vernon's acceptance of my presence. Peter doubted that he could adjust to having someone extra present in the room, if he needed assistance to be showered. In this, Peter imagined himself in Vernon's position. In imagining himself in Vernon's position, he acknowledged Vernon as a person, not just another patient subjected to a necessary routine. Peter thus acknowledged Vernon's uniqueness and his right to make choices about what felt acceptable for him.

Peter and Vernon interacted daily. They knew each other well enough to appreciate certain things about each other. Vernon appreciated Peter's straight talking, which motivated him, but he also acknowledged Peter's gentleness in coaxing him through his activities of daily living. Peter appreciated Vernon's courage to try to help himself. Peter loved Vernon's cheekiness and understood it for what it was; an older man tolerating his circumstances through a sense of fun.

Introducing William

William was born on 20 September, 1907. He has been living alone since his wife died in 1974. William experienced a cerebrovascular accident three years ago. He has been attending day care three times a week. Recently, he was admitted to hospital with a right fractured neck of femur, into which a dynamic hip screw has been inserted. William is rehabilitating in the PNU in preparation for going home. William prefers to be independent, stating that he 'doesn't want to be a burden', and he has agreed to stay with his son for a while after he leaves hospital.

Peter and William: a story about massage and motivation

Peter tells me he is ready to go to William to do a massage. As I walk down the corridor, a pre-registration nurse is asking Peter about the pain relief orders for William and they are discussing the strength and frequency of the various analgesics listed. I leave them while they go to get some Panadeine for William and tell them that I'll go to have a talk with him until they come. William is lying on his back in bed and when I greet him by name he calls me 'Bev.' I am surprised and elated that he remembers my name. I tell him Peter is on his way with some pain killers and that he will then do a massage. He is pleased.

Peter and the student nurse join us within minutes, and Peter gives the tablets to William and screens the bed. Peter tells William what he thinks he'll do and asks William whether he thinks it is better for him to lie face down or on his side. William says he'll leave that decision to Peter, so Peter says it might be best on his side and assists William to loosen and drop his trousers. The student nurse and I settle on the other side of the bed and Peter positions William on his left side and covers him ready for the massage. He will massage his left hip and thigh.

Peter checks that William is comfortable and begins the massage using mentholated oil. It is quiet. It is mid-afternoon outside and the traffic is light on the road outside the building. I can hear the faint voices of people on the street and there are some conversations between other people in this part of the building. It is a sleepy, overcast afternoon, and William is sleepy here, behind the curtain. Peter notices that William has his eyes closed, so Peter doesn't talk. He continues the massage in firm, long strokes and circular rubs.

Suddenly, after about three minutes, the quietness is broken by William. 'You have a good touch there!' he tells Peter. Peter replies with surprise: 'Oh, I thought you were asleep.' 'No, I'm awake. I can feel every move you make.' Peter checks that the massage is comfortable for him and he tells Peter that it is. Peter says that he feels William has had a bad day today and asks whether William wants to talk about it. William says that he felt 'very crook' this morning, because his leg has been hurting, but he doesn't move beyond a description of the physical uncomfortableness, before he shuts his eyes and relaxes again.

The massage continues for a few more minutes and Peter covers the exposed part with a towel and a wrap and asks William whether he'd like a sleep for a while. Bleary-eyed, William tells Peter he thinks he might have a nap. I tell William that I'll go too and come back later for a talk.

Interpretations

William was an ageing man with many cherished memories. He remembered his wife and recounted what happened on the day she died. He told me the story of his wife's death, because Peter's motivating force had reminded him of his wife's tendency to keep him pushing forwards towards their goals. William had suffered a lot of pain, due to his fractured hip, and his low emotional ebb meant that he was disinclined to push himself towards independence. He realised that Peter was trying to motivate him, to make him able to go home to live with his son, but he doubted that he could keep up his end of their bargain.

The nurse-patient interaction between William and Peter centred on Peter giving William a hip massage. When I analysed the text relating to the interaction between Peter and William, seven main qualities and activities emerged, which appeared to illuminate the phenomenon of ordinariness in nursing. The qualities and activities were: appreciating skilful nursing care; living with pain; approving commendable human qualities; talking straight; acknowledging the relevance of family affiliations; and relating to one another's humanness; acknowledging the importance of company and talking. These qualities and activities will be explained now.

Appreciating skilful nursing care. William appreciated the way in which Peter massaged his thigh and he was pleased generally with the nursing care in the PNU William said:

> 'It [the massage] was a nice feeling and the oil was soothing...It was very good...Yes, well he has got a good touch too. Yes, my word he has...It [the massage] was very similar to two or three I've had before. When he does it he puts a lot of strength in those hands. He's not just doing it, like, he puts some effort into it. I appreciate the service he gives and I always appreciate his manner...I think the nursing care is very good.'

Living with pain. William experienced pain in his hip and it was difficult for him to cope with it. He explained how Peter tried to help him cope with the pain and encouraged him to keep going about his daily activities.

> 'Yeah. It's a long while [three months] to put up with the pain, isn't it? Yes, yes, he's [Peter is] all for 'keep going.' He reckons that the results will be worth it. I still have my doubts. I don't agree with him all the way…I often tell him that the pain I go through is not worth it for the extra couple of years I might live.'

Peter knew that William was trying to bear the pain and he realised the effect that it was having on him. Peter said:

> 'I think the pain is [stopping William from walking more often]. It is getting him down. Pain becomes worse when you are depressed. It builds up and, although it may have started off as a slight pain, thinking about it constantly, depresses him more. He said to me the other night: "It is just wearing me down, wearing me down!"'

Approving commendable human qualities. William liked Peter's motivating nature, but William realised that he had to play an active part in his own recovery.

> 'He [Peter], as a man, I like him very much. He really is a very thoughtful sort of fellow. Yes. All I can say is that he's a good man. [crying]. I appreciate what he's trying to do…I've got to say that he'll never get anywhere without my ability too and I think it's too much for me to hold up my end.'

Peter had come to appreciate William's human qualities over the time he had been in the PNU.

> 'I think he's [William is] a nice man. When I first met him, he had a great sense of humour, but now he's not quite so lively as he was. He's got a lot of good stories to tell. He went down with the Canberra during the war on the Archangel convoys up to Russia. He's got a good few yarns to tell. He's an interesting man.'

Talking straight. William appreciated Peter's forthrightness in speaking clearly about what he thought was reasonable. William realised that Peter's straight talk helped him to keep on trying to help himself. He explained:

> 'He's [Peter has] got his own ideas about things though. As long as he thinks it's doing the job, well, well and good…He's got of a sort of 'stand over' manner. He thinks he's right and we are all entitled to our opinion. He thinks he's right and he goes ahead and does it. He knows sometimes you don't agree with him. Still, we don't fall out over that…I wouldn't like to see him change his manner…Well, I don't know, in the long run it might help me a lot. I could easily throw my hand in…He reckons it's worth it to keep going. He reckons the results are worth it.'

William explained how he and Peter would often interact when William experienced 'down days.'

[Laughs] 'He ignores me [on down days]! He'll let me rally on and then he'll say: "If you went home like this, what good are you to yourself? What can you do? Who will look after you?" I'll say: "If the worst comes to worst, I suppose I can have a go to a home or pay for help." He says: "That treatment may not come up to the standard you expect." [speaking as he laughs] Ye-ye-ye-ye-yes. No. he's a nice fellow."'

Relating to one another's humanness. William and Peter recognised each other as fellow human beings. William said:

'[I] can't understand how a man like him goes through life not married. [He] comes from around the midlands in England, where my wife came from...Yes. [starts to cry] He reminds me a lot of my Queenie, my wife...She's dead now. She had her ideas on life. She was a good woman, a good woman. Yes, he's a bit after her style.'

Peter recognised William's low mental ebb, as the present representation of William's humanness.

'He is very down and depressed and I am not too sure how we are going to get him up again.'

Acknowledging the relevance of family affiliations. When William said that Peter's nature reminded him of his wife, William told me the story of the events surrounding her death.

'Yes, Queenie wasn't her name, her name was Marigold. There were four boys in the family and when she was born, the eldest boy said: "We've got a little Queen at last!" Queenie stuck from there on...She was a good woman. I was lost when she went...It was '74, Christmas Eve...She was out at a nursing home...As I walked up towards the sister at the desk, she said: "Mr Connors, I'd like to speak to you (choking tears)". I was going to speak to her as a matter of courtesy, to say that I was visiting. I started to walk over to Queenie and she followed me and said: "Your wife passed away about a quarter of an hour ago". I said: "Good gawd! I've been sitting here on the verandah longer than that!" She said: "I'm very sorry, I didn't know you were out there." I asked her what happened. She said it was hard to know, but apparently it was her heart. Anyway, that was that!'

Peter realised that William's son was his nearest relative and that he meant a great deal to him. Peter was trying to prepare William for going home to be with his son. Peter explained:

'The way he [William] is depressed at the moment, he could end up going to a home or something...His son, yes. His son works, so he [William] will have to be reasonably independent, during the day at least.'

Acknowledging the importance of company and talking. Peter acknowledged the value of spending time and talking with people like William.

'Well, the reason I did the massage was that he [William] has been complaining about quite a lot of pain in his hip and knee and the other thing is, he is very depressed and I thought a little bit of human contact might help cheer him up a little bit. I was hoping to have the opportunity to let him talk about a few things, but he seemed to just be almost drifting off to sleep in a way, which is a good thing, I think. There's nothing wrong with that. You just have to go with the flow a bit. It was nice to have him relax and to know he feels it is of value.'

Peter felt that self disclosure was therapeutic in interpersonal relationships with patients. He said:

'I can't see any reason [why you should not tell patients about yourself]. You expect them to tell you about themselves. Why shouldn't we [nurses] reciprocate? All the textbooks on [psycho-analytic] therapeutic communication say that your background is of no interest to the patient.'

Peter also acknowledged the value of general conversation with patients.

'Also, always concentrating on their [patients'] problems and things like that, that gets a bit wearing for both the staff and the patient, I think. Like, sometimes a general conversation, about nothing in particular, about things that happen in the paper, things that happen in the world, your history, or anything like that, just like normally, if you met someone in the pub or at a coffee shop or something like that. Why do you have to be focussing on some particular [illness] aspect? I think conversation is just a—like it is a distraction as well. If you are in pain, it is a way of distracting you from pain and...'

Conclusions

William had a long and painful stay in hospital. At first it was thought that he did not have a fractured hip, but eventually it was diagnosed, so he had at least three months in almost constant pain. Peter had lived through William's long hospitalisation experience with him and he had used massage, encouragement and analgesics, to relieve as much of William's pain as he possibly could.

Peter also knew William's stories of war time. He thought William was an interesting man and he remembered a time before the pain, when William had a sense of humour. Peter shared some of himself with William. He joked that his life has been nowhere near as interesting as William's, but he shared it, for what it is worth. Peter expressed the idea that it was reasonable for nurses to disclose something of themselves to patients, otherwise there was an imbalance in their relationship. Peter valued general conversation between nurses and patients, because day to day life was also about light talk and common interests.

Peter was working with William to get him home to his son. He was trying to help William to be as independent as possible, but he feared that William's depression might result ultimately in him being transferred to a nursing home, rather than to William's son's home, where he preferred to go.

William appreciated Peter's manner; he likened it to that of his deceased wife. She had a strong will and encouraged him to keep going and William saw something of her in Peter. Thinking of his wife sparked the memory of her death on Christmas Eve in 1974. As he recounted the story, the pain was as fresh as ever. He cried for her as he told the story. It gave him pain, but he wanted to talk about her, because Peter had a similar style of encouraging him to do things.

William resigned himself to the idea that he might end up in the same nursing home, in which his wife died. He knew, when he encouraged him, that Peter was only concerned with his welfare. William appreciated what Peter was trying to do to help him, but he recognised his own part in his recovery and he was unsure that he could keep up his end of the bargain in trying to gain relative independence.

7. Sally's nurse-patient interactions

Introducing Sally

Sally became a nurse when she was eighteen years and three months old and she has been nursing for ten years. Sally always wanted to be a nurse, but she doesn't know why, except that she thinks she 'probably picked up on other people thinking that [she] cared for people well, so for [her] it was just a natural progression.' For Sally nursing is about 'being able to make a difference for someone, maybe to give them a bit of their confidence back, either to adapt to what's happened to them, or to help them understand what's happening to them.' She lets them know what the options are, for them to understand at their own level. Sally's hopes for her own future in nursing include working in community nursing, such as district nursing, or a day hospital, or a hospice organisation. The hope Sally holds for nursing itself in the future is that it will go much more into the community and get away from rule-ridden hospital settings. She feels that 'in small places you are more likely to have multiprofessional teams sitting around talking together, whereas in a hospital setting there is a definite hierarchal setting, which is hard to avoid.'

Introducing Frances

Frances was born on 6 July 1910. She lives at home with her husband. She was admitted to the PNU recently after a mild cerebrovascular accident. She was at the point at which she needed motivation, in getting herself back into her usual routines of daily living.

Sally and Frances: a story about negotiating independence

It is about 10.15 p.m. Sally, the night nurse, is making her rounds with her drug trolley, settling people for the night. Frances has been waiting until Sally gets to her. Sally greets her and asks her about her day. Sally consults the drug chart to prepare the tablets. Sophie, the other night nurse, whispers to Frances to suggest a pan. Sally says she has good hearing and reminds Frances that she thinks it would be a good idea if she sits on a commode to empty her bladder thoroughly and then she may have fewer awakenings through the night.

Frances remembers a discussion she had with Sally previously and Sophie goes to get the commode. The bed is screened and Sophie helps Frances out of bed and assists her to guide herself onto the commode. The urination over, Frances gets back into bed and settles to take the tablets Sally has prepared for her.

When Frances is comfortably back in bed, Sally spends some time talking with her about her drugs and her progress generally. It is time spent with her exclusively, even though time is passing and we are still in the first room. Sophie is standing at the drug trolley. She looks at me and tells me that the time they spend now is worthwhile. She compares Sally with other night nurses and says the others tend to rush through this round and often the patients seem less settled. Sally hears what is being said and she affirms her opinion that it is time well spent.

Sally talks with Frances for about five minutes. They had talked before about some concerns Frances has and this conversation reviews and affirms the decisions they made together then. Frances looks settled and talks easily with Sally, who takes her time to be with her.

The time has come to say goodnight to everyone in this room. There is quiet in the room and some of the women are already slumbering. The four women in this room are settled and the main room light is turned out and with a final wish of 'Goodnight,' Sally, Sophie, and I move to the next room.

Interpretations

Frances was recovering from a stroke and she was trying to regain her independence. Sally and Frances had discussed a strategy for assisting Frances towards independence, that of using a night time commode before settling. On this particular occasion, Frances asked for a pan and Sally reminded her of the plan they had negotiated previously.

I analysed the text relating to the interaction between Sally and Frances and eight main qualities and activities emerged, which were: appreciating skilful nursing care; approving commendable human qualities; valuing the patient as person; valuing the nurse as person; facilitating coping; acknowledging the importance of company and talking; relating to the other's hummanness and building trust.

Appreciating skilful nursing care. Frances appreciated the time Sally spent with her preparing her for sleep and negotiating with her a method of night toileting. She said:

> [Sally is] wonderful. She really made you happy and gave you the best class of care you could have, you know, and something for the pain. I had one [a tablet] to help me sleep and I slept right through. She fixes you up and gets you up in bed and that. She's wonderful...Yes, but it [using a commode] was hard. Everything's hard, but she said it was better not having the pan in the bed and having the exercise, and the toilet is too far to go to, and so they got me onto that. But this morning I had to go down to the toilet. See, when you've got waterworks trouble, it's terrible, isn't it?'

Approving commendable human qualities. Frances was appreciative of Sally's qualities.

> 'She's very kind and speaks nicely to you and to help you, you know. Nothing's a trouble to her. She's very good, very good. She's capable and she's pleasant. Marvellous...Oh, she is, she's excellent. I would like to take her home with me. Yes, I really would. And she's always got a kind word and that does make a difference, doesn't it...But she is, she is a very sweet person. And she's got such a personality with everyone. A little pat and that, you know. It makes you feel good. She is excellent. Well, they all are, but of course I haven't been here so long to know so much about it. She [Sally] never complains. She says: "Well, if the bell doesn't ring we'd just have our heads down on the table and we'd be nearly asleep and we can't afford to go to sleep." Keep her awake!!'. (Laugh)

Frances commended the other nurses also.

> 'She's [Sally is] excellent, she really is, they all are as a matter of fact. And the little girl [Sophie, the other night nurse], who goes around with Sally, she's so kind. She has such a lovely face. She always has a kind word. A kind word is so much better that a harsh one isn't it? Well, I suppose they wouldn't be nurses if they weren't kind. Although I remember I have met unkind nurses...They treat you like you're unreal, don't they? Well, no one wants to be sick, no one wants to be here [in hospital].'

Valuing the patient as person. Frances felt that Sally treated her as though she was a person. Frances explained:

> 'Yes, you feel as though you are a person. You're not just rushed, you know, with a pill. She talks about odds and ends you know, where you've got the pain and about the feeling and that. All the night nurses are good, but I find her very special.'

Valuing the nurse as person. In addition to being treated as a person by Sally, Frances sensed Sally's humanness.

'I think she's very human, you know. [Sally] tells you: "Everybody's going through it, you know, and don't throw the sponge in!" Cause I said to her the other night [begins to cry] "I may as well be dead. "'

Facilitating coping. Frances and Sally planned together to help Frances cope generally by becoming more independent following her stroke. Sally described Frances' problem.

'A week ago, when she [Frances] first came in, she couldn't do certain things; she couldn't get out of bed and walk as far down the hallway and now she can, so it was just something positive for her to look back and say: "Well, yeah, even if I am feeling miserable, things are getting better". It was really a big dependent thing. When I pulled the curtain shut, that's another thing I talked about with her, her embarrassment on the pan. I said: "Well, let's start getting over hurdles to build your confidence up."'

Frances disliked seeking help. She explained:

'Because I hate ringing the bell. I feel as if I'm causing trouble.'

Sally tried to dispel Frances' concern about seeking help. She said:

'So I just sort of spent some time and said: "At least being in here, you don't have to ask us. We can be there to offer before you feel you need to ask."'

Frances tried using the commode at night, but remained fairly unconvinced of the value of it. Frances said:

'But you know, I think a bedpan's better [than the commode], well it's easier anyway. If you're careful you never make a mistake.'

However, Frances knew that Sally's suggestions were well-intentioned.

'Well, they (Sally and Sophie) are all doing it for a reason, you know, and you know they are doing it to help you, because they know they can't be home with you all the time and if you want to go home, well you've got to do these things.'

Sally explained how she felt it would help Frances, if she could become accustomed to using a commode.

'So I thought it [getting out of bed onto a commode] would help her two-fold: get the physical movements back to scratch and get her feeling less embarrassed or less dependent on us. She can get out and we can come back when she's finished. Then it will be a natural progression from needing a pan before, to using a commode, building on what she can do.'

When Frances appeared to be accepting the offer of a pan from Sophie, Sally reminded Frances of their agreement.

'Tonight I said: "We talked about this [the benefits of using a commode]. I'm not going to let you forget about his. We are going to keep working on this." I had said to her: "Tonight we will start and we will use the commode." I didn't know whether she was trying to get away without getting out on a commode, or whether she had forgotten. I piped up and gave her an opportunity to say either: "I was in a real hurry and I needed to go straight away" or "I forgot". Yes, we did talk about that.'

Acknowledging the importance of company and talking. The dialogue between Sally and Frances had been ongoing over several occasions. Talking together made it possible to plan some independence strategies for Frances. Sally explained:

'Well, what happened tonight [reminding Frances about the use of the commode] stemmed from something that happened this morning. It was about half past five in the morning or thereabouts and she'd had a pan and she was really upset and she's made a comment to Sophie actually and I thought "Oh, hang on, I'm not sure about that," so I went back in to talk with her and she just about burst into tears. I talked to her about it and she explained what it was that she was worried about. Her tone and her face changed while I was there for that ten minutes.'

Relating to the other's humanness. Sally understood Frances' need to be independent, because she needed to be independent also.

'She (Frances) said: "I'm so used to helping other people, that I'm not used to them helping me." I can relate to that, because I'm pretty independent too and don't like other people doing things I could do myself.'

Building trust. Sally expressed the need to follow through on a negotiated plan, in order to build trust.

'I thought "Slow down Sophie, you're getting in front of me. That was something I wanted to do [settle Frances for the night]". Yes [you have to follow through on a plan], otherwise it doesn't carry any weight and they don't know whether they can trust you, because you've told them one thing and you didn't follow through with it.'

Conclusions

Frances was trying to become as independent as possible and she disclosed this need to Sally. Together they planned some strategies for building Frances' confidence, and one idea was for Frances to get out of bed to use the commode on settling, in preparation for using one when she went home. They decided that using a commode at night would also give Frances some independence, exercise, and confidence in helping herself generally.

That evening on settling time, however, Frances indicated to the other night nurse, who was working with Sally, that she would like to use a pan in bed. Sophie was not aware of the arrangement and offered her a pan. Sally intervened and reminded Frances of the pact to use the commode. Frances agreed to use the commode and Sophie helped her out of bed to use it. Although Frances expressed a preference for the using a pan, she was willing to persevere with the commode, given that she and Sally had already discussed the reasons for this decision.

Her part in giving the pact a chance to be successful, was important to Sally. She felt that if she did not follow through in encouraging Frances with the plan, that Frances would lose her trust in their relationship. It was important to Sally that she built trust with Frances. She encouraged Frances by reminding her of their previous discussion and making it as easy as possible for the commode to be used the first time it was tried.

Frances expressed her need to be as independent as possible and together she and Sally planned some strategies. Frances appreciated what Sally was trying to do and even though it meant considerable effort, with Sally's continued encouragement, she persevered with the plan to use the commode. Frances appreciated the way in which Sally treated her as a person and the humanness Sally displayed in her work. Together, they worked as a team, building trust and confidence.

Introducing Gus

Gus was born on 15 April 1908. He lives at home with his wife, having retired to town from their country property. Gus was admitted to the PNU after an above knee amputation for peripheral vascular disease and a leg ulcer, which resulted, and persisted, from a lack of blood supply. Gus is now at the stage of being up and about the unit in his wheelchair and during the day he keeps himself busy trying to learn to stand on his unaffected leg, so that he can get the stage of being ready for a prosthetic leg fitting.

Sally and Gus: a story about phantom pain

Gus is in the corridor near the entrance to the unit; he likes to stay there to practise sitting and standing on his right leg. His left leg is amputated above the knee because of peripheral vascular disease and a painful leg ulcer, which persisted for years. But now he is without the leg and without the ulcer, and he is getting accustomed to the phantom pain and to life with one leg. He spends the day in his wheelchair and wheels himself away from the main traffic of the unit, to the far end of the corridor, to practice standing and sitting at the walking rails attached to the walls. By night, his favourite spots in the unit are the sitting room and the front entrance. He doesn't like the nights; they are long and it is a time when his leg 'plays up.'

He is a slightly built old man. He wears thick, black-rimmed spectacles, which have a piece of cotton wadding on the rim above his eyes to make the glasses less heavy on his brow. His small round face is kind, and his hair is sparse, giving him an appearance not unlike Foo. He is hard of hearing and his hearing aid is non-functioning at present. He wheels himself around listening to his Walkman audiotapes and loves to spend time talking with anyone who'll have a chat with him.

Tonight, he has agreed to participate in my study, and Sally tells me they will go to the sunroom for a chat before he is ready to go to bed. She tells me that he has fallen asleep at the front entrance and she doesn't want to wake him. She is concerned that it is late and that I might be inconvenienced. I tell her I'm happy to wait and that if Gus wants to go straight to bed when he awakens from his slumber, we can talk another time. About ten minutes passes and I go to prepare myself a mug of coffee. Gus is not at the entrance of the unit. We walk towards his room and we meet him as he is coming out. He is happy to have a chat and a drink. He doesn't want to settle yet.

We go to the sitting room and sit down. Gus has a drink of Milo, that Sally has prepared for him. Sally tells him she would like to talk about how he will manage on his weekend leave. He tells her the occupational therapist was not keen for him to stay away for more than two days, because the house hasn't been adapted, but that his wife has insisted that they will be quite alright.

The conversation is at top volume, because he is deaf and his aid is not working at present. When Sally wants to talk she must lean forward and speak into his right ear. It is late and Sally looks drawn. She told me earlier that she has a headache and it seems as though it might still be there.

Gus is in a talking mood and he sails into a description of his farming life in the Mallee and of his days on the Murray with the paddle boats. He talks for about fifteen minutes non-stop. He has 'fair dinkum Aussie' language and a bush humour I recognise. He talks with great absorption in his topic and barely stops for breath. Sally is looking pale. Gus keeps on talking.

Eventually, she stands up and leans in to him and tells him she has a headache. Gus thinks he has caused the headache and he apologises. She tries to tell him that she had it before, but he can't hear her and she has to repeat herself three or four times. She looks like she is about to give up trying to have him understand, because of the effort of making him hear. He keeps on talking, so she puts her fingers in front of her lips and says 'Ssh, ssh.' He sees and he stops talking. She tells him she has to go, because she is not feeling well. He understands and he nods. She gives me a half smile and leaves the room. I thank her and approach Gus to begin our talk.

Interpretations

Eight main qualities and activities emerged when I analysed the text relating to the interaction between Sally and Gus, using the method that I have described previously in Chapter 2. The qualities and activities were: acknowledging the importance of company and talking; acknowledging the importance of home and family; approving commendable human qualities; relating to one another's humanness; enjoying a sense of humour; expressing affection and liking; relating to one another's situation; and expressing feelings.

Acknowledging the importance of company and talking. Gus acknowledged the importance of company and talk. At night, his phantom pain was worse and he survived the early morning hours, knowing that Sally and Sophie were there to be with him. Gus said:

> 'Well, myself, I found it [the conversation with Sally] good. I mean to say, she's a busy girl and I could talk to her all day and all night. Do you know what I mean? Well, they'll [the nurses will] do anything for you, to help you. Anytime. I could sit here all night and I'd still get my cups of tea or coffee and all that. They'd come in at night time, 'cause I'd be in trouble at night time. I used to prop that [the amputated leg] and make a noise some nights. They'd hear me, and they'd come in and say: "I don't think that this [the phantom pain] can be fixed. It's gotta just take its own course, I think."'

Gus knew that the painkillers were ineffective and there was nothing else Sally could do, but to be with him. Gus continued:

> 'They could do nothing to help me really, but they'd come up and I'd get a cup of coffee and something to eat as the case might be and that sort of help.

*And if I wanted any help again, I'd get it. If I made a noise or pressed the
button, they'd be there again. But, I enjoy their company, you know.'*

Sally acknowledged the importance of being with Gus during the
night.

'It was just a bit of a chat, because there's not a lot that we actually
do physically, or whatever, with him at night. So, it's to let him
know that we have time for him, even though we are not necessarily
doing a task.'

Sally related the story of one night, which was particularly
horrendous for Gus and how her presence helped. Gus had been
on weekend leave and returned to the PNU Sally explained:

'One of his nights was terrific ['terrifically awful']. I mean he talks
about 'nights,' because that's when he gets his phantom pain. He
had one good night [at home], probably the best he's ever had.
The next night was really miserable and he was up all night with
the phantom pain, which flared up worse than it had been for a
long time. Consequently, his first night back in here, which was
last night, he was miserable and there was nothing we could do
apart from being around, so that he could talk to us if he wanted
to; you know, just our presence. I don't think I've seen him that
bad. He's got a headphone tape player [the batteries had gone flat
but I changed them for new ones] and he didn't even want to know
about it. He said: "I've got to get up, I've got to get up!" He got up
and went to the TV room, where he proceeded to go off to sleep.
    I think he is very conscious of disturbing other people [in his
room]. He gets upset thinking he's bothering other people. He's a
lot brighter tonight. Just sort of being there for him, we've tried
rubs, hot packs and chemical analgesics, and all sorts of things, but
nothing really works. He said to Sophie [the other night nurse] last
night. "I know it's all in here [indicating his head], but the pain is
right there [pointing to his missing limb]. I know it should be getting
better, but it's there and it hurts."'

Acknowledging the importance of home and family. Gus was
a keen story teller and many of his yarns related to his life on his
farm in the Murray River region. Gus's love of home and family
were inextricably bound to his identity as a person. Gus said:

*'About the farm. Well, ah, let me put it this way. I can't bring myself to
be a city lad. I've always been a country boy. And that's all there is to it.
You might have seen the movie picture All the Rivers Run. I have the
book at home and it's a true book, and all the river boats mentioned in
that book are true. I don't know them all, because at the time there was
about one hundred boats hanging around Echuca. But only a few came
up[stream] to us; the Lachlan, the Murrumbidgee and the Darling and
the Edwards. Well, that's all about I can say. Then there were the
passenger boats the Ruby and the Jenny.'*

Gus expressed his adoration of the nurses, but he was careful to prioritise his wife at the top of his list of 'sweethearts.'

'I've got a wonderful wife and a wonderful lot of girls [emotional] between here and my wife. I've got a lot of sweethearts. (Laugh) But my wife's on top. Don't forget that! (Laugh)'

Approving commendable human qualities. Gus was full of praise for the commendable human qualities he recognised in Sally, Sophie and the other nurses.

'Well, to be candid, I think she's [Sally is] a beautiful girl, because she's so kind in every way to me, since I've been here. Never been any different. And, I know I'm an old bloke, but still, I love these girls here. And, to be honest with you, from the time I was in hospital from the first time, from the time to here, I've struck every nurse as a wonderful nurse. They'd do anything for me. I don't know why.'

Sally acknowledged that Gus encouraged them in caring for him as they did. Sally said:

'Well, he's good. He constantly gives us compliments and praise, which is really nice.'

Relating to one another's humanness. Gus considered himself to be nothing terribly special in himself and he was in awe of the care he received from the nurses.

'I'm nothing special. I'm just an old man. (Laugh). But, oh Jees, you know. Oh, I try to be [good company for them too], even if some times I wonder whether I am or not. (giggle).'

The night she interacted with Gus, Sally had a severe headache. She struggled to listen to Gus as he told his stories, but she was unable to bear the pain. Even though she enjoyed his company, Sally had to acknowledge her own human needs for space and quietness.

'Well, Gus is very hard of hearing; I mean he's deaf. You've got to shout and even then he doesn't necessarily understand what you are saying. I had taken him down to a room, where we could close the door and block out some of the noise we were going to create by talking. We got comfortable and he just started to chat and he wasn't going to stop chatting, story after story. I'd take a big breath and think "I will get in here," but I couldn't.
I also happened to have a throbbing headache that night, and because I had to speak louder to get him to hear me, and because he was booming, it just sort of made me feel worse. I thought "This isn't a positive interaction." I sat the time out for while. A couple of times, I actually sat forward in the chair and tried to cut in and I couldn't do it. There just wasn't a chance.'

Enjoying a sense of humour. Gus enjoyed the sense of fun he shared with the nurses.

'As I say, I have a lot of fun with them. I know I'm a bit cheeky sometimes, but I have a lot of fun with them.'

Expressing affection and liking. Gus's feelings for the night nurses extended past respect for their human qualities. He liked them as people, who he regarded as his friends.

'Well, look here, really and truly, the night nurses, I couldn't speak highly enough of them. That's putting it plain. All the nurses here in the day time are good. I sort of wait for these girls of a night time. I know the night will be long and I've got to go through it and they get here [to the PNU] about nine o'clock I think and I may be just a stupid old bloke, but I just sort of look forward to seeing them coming in at night time. I think they are bonza girls, that's what I think. They are lovely and I love the whole bloomin' lot. The night nurses, Sophie and this one [Sally], I love them both, because they are good girls, lovely girls.'

Relating to one another's situation. Sally felt ambivalent initially about telling Gus about her headache, because she knew how much he loved to talk.

'It was like "I really wish I wasn't here." I thought I could get through it and when I was sitting there and listening to him I thought "It is really awful, because I don't want to be here. I can't concentrate properly and appreciate his stories," because he tells wonderful stories.'

When Sally finally managed to tell Gus about her headache, he felt for her pain. Sally said:

'He sort of told me to go off and have some Panadol and make sure that I was alright and that I should look after myself and he continued to apologise. Well, I think the message got across [that he didn't cause my headache], but I think that he realised that if he had a headache and someone was shouting at him [it wouldn't be too nice]…It was probably because he could put himself in my shoes.'

Expressing feelings. Even though it was difficult to overcome her ambivalence about telling Gus about her headache, Sally knew that she had to express her feelings to Gus to be honest with him about how she was feeling at that time.

'So, I managed to jump in at one stage and explain to him that I wasn't feeling well and then of course he got all upset, because he thought he'd caused my headache, and I felt really miserable, because I didn't want him to think that he'd caused it, but to just let him know that because of it I'd had to cut our time short. I managed to get around that and I did leave, but after that particular time, I went back to him and helped him into bed and explained to him that I'd had a headache before I'd even seen him and that it was just me thinking I would give it a try and that I could probably manage.'

Sally felt that it was important to express to Gus how her headache was making her feel.

'Well, I can't see the point in hiding that [the headache], because I started to fidget when my head was really hurting and I wanted to get out. I thought "I can't just get up and walk out." That's not me, but I just got so uncomfortable…I apologised later for cutting him off, because I do find his stories interesting. He said: "Yes, but I could tell you stories all night!" He's a talker.'

Conclusions

Gus was recovering from an above knee amputation and he was experiencing a great deal of pain, especially at night. He found the evenings most difficult to bear, because it was then that his phantom pain was at its worst. Gus looked forward to Sally and Sophie coming on duty, because he knew they would be there with him, as he rode out the phantom pain. Sally felt they were powerless to alleviate Gus's pain, other than to supply the usual analgesics, tea and talk.

Gus loved to talk. Sally and Gus often talked before he settled. The conversations were usually at top volume, because Gus was deaf and his hearing aid was not working. On this particular evening, Gus was in a talking mood and he sailed into a description of his farming life in the Mallee and of his days on the Murray with the paddle boats. He talked with great absorption in his topic and barely stopped for breath. Sally was looking pale, but Gus kept on talking.

That evening, Sally had a headache and although she tried to stay with Gus and remain interested in his stories, she knew that she was physically unable to listen this time. She was undergoing inner turmoil knowing that he loved to talk and that, usually, she liked to listen, but she was having difficulty finding a break in Gus's talking to explain to him what was happening for her. She waited at least fifteen minutes, before she told Gus that she had a headache.

Gus thought that he had caused the headache and he apologised. She tried to tell him that she had the headache before their conversation, but he couldn't hear her and she had to repeat herself three or four times. She looked like she was about to give up trying to have him understand, because of the effort of making him hear. He kept on talking so she put her fingers in front of her lips and said: 'Ssh, ssh.' He stopped talking and she told him she had to go, because she was not feeling well. He understood and he nodded to her.

When she was finally able to explain her headache to him, he thought he had caused it and it was not till later that they were able to clear up the misunderstanding. Gus knew he was a talker and Sally realised that he ultimately felt sorry for her, when he suggested she have some rest and pain killers. Gus and Sally truly cared for each other.

In his stories of appreciation, Gus referred to 'the nurses,' always including Sophie, because Sally and Sophie worked as a team on night duty. They all understood one another. He was bearing the phantom pain and they were helping him through the experience with tea, talk and company, because they knew that Gus's pain was real. There was nothing else they could do, but than to rid Gus of the night phantom by seeing him through his experience, by being there with him.

Introducing Beryl

Beryl was born on 12 March 1907. She lives locally with her daughter. Beryl was admitted to the PNU recently for some assistance in managing her pulmonary oedema and rheumatoid arthritis.

Sally and Beryl: a story about settling for the night

It is about 10 p.m. and Sally, the night nurse, is moving from person to person helping to settle them for the night. In a four bed room, Beryl is lying on her back. She does not have her teeth in. When Sally goes to her, Beryl covers her mouth to talk. Sally crouches down beside her to head height and talks with her about the drugs she is due to have now. They talk together quietly while Sophie (the other night nurse) continues to settle the women at the other side of the room.

Beryl has pulmonary oedema, yet she chooses to lie flat at night. At first Sally thinks Beryl is self-medicating, so she takes her tray of pills over to Beryl. She realises that Beryl has not begun her self-medicating practice yet, so she takes time to tell her what each drug is for, before she offers them to Beryl.

They then talk about Beryl's palpitations, which sometimes trouble her at night. Sally explains that it is related to her chest problem. Sally suggests that if she gets breathless during the night, that Beryl could sit up and she tells her that many people who have her condition prefer to sleep sitting up. Beryl says she likes to sleep lying down, but listens to what Sally is saying. She takes her tablets and remains lying on her back. Every now and then Beryl remembers that she doesn't have her teeth in and gives a coy smile and covers her mouth. Sally does not make a fuss about Beryl's gummy mouth, but continues to talk softly with her.

When the conversation is over, Sally stands up and prepares a drink to help Beryl take the pills. Beryl takes the pills Sally has dispensed and settles down in bed again. As Sally moves away, Beryl is already looking sleepy.

Interpretations

Beryl was a lonely woman, because she had just been admitted to the nursing unit and, as to date, she had not created a friendship with anyone. Beryl waited for her daughter to visit and was thrilled to have her daughter's friends visit her also. Sally was only just beginning to get to know Beryl when she talked with her, as she helped to settle her for the night. On this occasion of nursing care, Sally talked to Beryl about relieving some of her night time dyspnoea and palpitations, by sitting up leaning on pillows to sleep.

When I analysed the text relating to the interaction between Sally and Beryl seven main qualities and activities emerged, which were: appreciating skilful nursing care; approving commendable human qualities; acknowledging the importance of company and talking; expressing feelings; acknowledging the relevance of family affiliations; facilitating changes; and taking time to know one another.

Appreciating skilful nursing care. Beryl was impressed with the way in which Sally gave her explanations about her heart and therapy. Beryl said:

> 'Well, she explained the pumping of my heart. It seems to come from my back, when I was lying down and she said if I felt like that, it would be best to either sit up or put an extra pillow, because I like to lie very flat. She said that could ease the pumping, you know. It's not a pumping really, it's just the heart beats seem to go quicker, heavier...Yes I am more aware of it than I am usually. I am more aware of it when it does that. You know, it starts to 'kind of' beating heavier and it seems to come right from my back. What it is, I don't know, but this is it. She explained to me what could ease me if I wanted, if it came on again, which is very good of her...Well, she explains everything so's I have detail. I mean she tells me what my pills are I'm having, she just tells me each one—not that I can remember, but she tells me each one I'm having—what they are for, which is nice to know what you're going to get. She explains things so clearly and tells me what every pill is.'

Approving commendable human qualities. Beryl liked Sally for various qualities she saw in her.

'I thought she was very nice and I liked her very much. She's a lovely girl! Well, she's so gentle. She's so gentle, well they all are. Sally seems to explain things [Beryl then tells her daughter about the pumping]. She's so helpful, she tells me what every pill is about and explains everything to me, you know. She is really marvellous.'

Beryl approved of all the nurses.

'Anyway, I rather liked Sally, she is nice nurse. Well, I don't know if she's a nurse, sister, or what. Yes. I call them all sisters. Oh, everybody's been wonderful. This is my third ward and everybody has been wonderful to me, they've done everything they can for me.'

Beryl also approved of other unit staff.

'Well, they are all nice. Even the cleaner comes and has a little chat to me. They're great.'

Acknowledging the importance of company and talking. Beryl had just moved from another ward to the PNU, into a room which she did not like, because she missed the company of the previous patients. She explained:

'Well, this ward...can I be honest? You see, one of the other patients in the other ward I was in, used to come to talk to me and I could talk to her. Now, I've tried talking to that lady [indicating to her right] and she can't hear what I'm saying. I can't understand that lady [indicating a German woman] and that lady [adjacent] doesn't seem to talk to anyone, so it's like, more or less...the other ward the patients talked to one another, whereas here I'm just on my own. I don't mind being on my own, I'm a lonely person really in that way, but, sometimes it does feel nice if you could just have a little conversation with the next patient who's with you. But in here you can't. I just wait for my daughter coming in.'

We talked about Beryl's future options for securing company and talk. I suggested that Elizabeth could probably arrange for Beryl to go and sit with some other women, who could talk English and could hear her, so that she would not be lonely. Beryl replied:

'I'm a poor mixer, unless they mix with me. I'm alright once I know them, but I can't push. When I came down here I was going to get on my feet and there was a television room and a games room and everything, but, it was going to be great down there, I could sit down there, but I haven't had the pleasure yet, to get down there.'

Expressing feelings. Beryl was tearful that day. She had tried too hard to mobilise herself and was feeling tired and weepy. She said:

'Yes, well, when I get on my feet [I'll go up to the television room]. This morning I had a very bad set back. I've had one of those weepy days today.'

Sally expressed her surprise when Beryl related her story of that day. Sally was given a night report with which Beryl's comments did not tally at first.

> 'What struck me first with her was when I first said: "How was your day?" She denied overdoing it or anything. But then she said: "Oh, well, I have been sort of pushing myself a bit. It was my own fault." Maybe she thought I meant "Did the nurses work you too hard today?" Then, when she had a think about it, she said: "No." She had pushed herself too far. I don't know whether it was the look on my face or if my voice had a bit of disbelief, like "Are you sure there's not something else?" But she's a lovely old lady.'

Acknowledging the relevance of family affiliations. Beryl valued her daughter's company and was touched that her daughter's friends also came to visit her. Beryl explained her weepiness to her daughter.

> *'I had a shower today, but I had to be wheeled. I tried to be clever yesterday and did too much.'*

Facilitating changes. Sally spent time explaining the benefits of sleeping semi-upright, however, Beryl preferred to remain lying down and Sally did not impose the change of position on her.

> 'Yes, well that's what I was trying to get her to sit up, but I don't know that she was aware of [the benefits of] sitting up…Yes, because if she can sleep and is comfortable sleeping that way [lying down], it's going to override anything else, because that's how she likes to sleep.'

Taking time to know one another. Sally acknowledged that it would take time to get to know Beryl's idiosyncrasies. In talking about Beryl's shyness in conversing without her dentures, Sally tried to be as sensitive as possible to how Beryl was feeling.

> 'Yes, I just told her I'd turn my head away or pretend that she had her teeth in. Yes, that was only the second time I've met her, so it's still getting to know what she needs.'

Conclusions

Beryl had only just been transferred to the PNU and the relative shortness of her stay, the severity of her condition, and the mix of people in her room, meant that she was missing the benefits of company. Beryl waited for her daughter to visit and she was touched when her daughter's friends came to visit her also. All in all, Beryl was feeling sad and lonely.

Sally interacted with Beryl as she prepared her for a night's sleep. Beryl experienced palpitations and when Sally dispensed her drugs, she gave Beryl some reasons why this might be so. Sally connected Beryl's experience of palpitations to her heart attempting to beat harder against strain and suggested that it might be relieved in part by Beryl sitting up to sleep.

Although Sally had given Beryl a logical reason for sitting up, Beryl remained lying flat in bed. Sally offered Beryl an option if she found that her breathing became more difficult and did not impose the upright position on Beryl. Sally allowed her to make her own choice, because lying down to sleep was what Beryl preferred. In allowing Beryl the right to make a choice about how she would sleep, Sally acknowledged that Beryl was living her own experience of her condition, in the way she understood.

Beryl had been 'weepy' yesterday and today and she put it down to having pushed herself too hard. Beryl accepted that she felt weepy for the time being and she appreciated Sally's gentleness, niceness and explanations; all of which were very important to her at that time.

8. Sue's nurse-patient interactions

Introducing Sue

Sue recalls that when she was ten years old, she had her tonsils out. A little girl across the way, who wasn't coping with her tonsillectomy, was crying so she started holding her hand. When she was eighteen, Sue made a decision to become a nurse, instead of a teacher. Sue began her nurse training in 1973, when she was twenty years old. Sue believes that 'caring is the central ingredient' of nursing and that nursing is about the ability to care for someone and their family unit. For Sue, nursing is a matter of giving of herself, sharing herself quite openly with a patient and also working in close conjunction with her peers. What Sue loves about nursing is being 'a bedside nurse' and what she hates is the paper work. In the future, Sue has a dream of setting up an Oncology Unit, as a nursing unit. The hopes she holds for nursing in the future are that 'nursing units and primary nursing will become much more accepted across the board' and that nurses will begin to make some changes to medical dominance.

Introducing Becky

Becky was born on 14 October 1925. She lives at home with her husband, who offers no domestic help. Becky had an oophorectomy and hysterectomy for menorrhagia, at thirty-eight years of age, after which she was not given oestrogen replacement. Becky is now presenting with fractured ribs from osteoporosis and she has been admitted to the PNU for mobilisation and also for help to ease her depression.

Sue and Becky: a story about relieving pain

Becky is ready for her bath. Sue has taken her clean clothes to the bathroom and she has selected some oils to put into the bath. Becky walks beside her to the bathroom. She is short of stature, stooped slightly forward. She is wearing a pink dressing gown, that is pulled firmly around her thin waist. Her face is etched with lines and her expression is one of tiredness with discomfort. Sue tells me that Becky has been vomiting this morning and that she had a restless night. We walk quietly together to the bathroom and shut the door.

Becky sits down on a chair and begins to undress herself. She tells me she is independent and that she would like to do as much as she can herself now. I tell her to let me know if I can help her. She gives me her dressing gown to hang on the peg behind the door. Sue half fills the bath with warm water and adds a few drops of each of the oils, naming each one and explaining what they are for. She tells Becky that they are for pain and anxiety relief and that there is one to make her feel happy. Then she shakes in some Radox crystals and the aroma of oils fills the bathroom.

Becky is undressed and Sue assists her into the bath. Becky's movements are slow and deliberate and Sue waits for her to set the pace. Becky settles into the bath and Sue shows her where the buzzer is and tells her to ring it when she is ready to get out, or if she needs her for anything. We leave Becky in the aroma of the oils and go to make her bed.

About ten minutes later, Sue calls me and I join Sue and Becky in the bathroom. Becky is looking relaxed and tells Sue she will pull herself up. She turns herself in the bath to orient herself to the side-rail with her strong arm. She tells us that she can't pull herself up with her other arm. Sue jokes that she wouldn't be able to turn herself sideways in a bath like that, because she is too tall and too large generally. Becky pulls herself upright and accepts Sue's arm to step over the side of the bath. Sue puts a towel on the floor and tells Becky that no one falls over with her, because she is almost six foot tall.

Becky is concentrating on getting out of the bath, but she gives a slight smile at Sue's comments. Becky takes a towel and wipes herself before wrapping it around her body and sitting on a towel Sue has placed in the chair. Becky continues to wipe her body and Sue hands her her Lily of the Valley talcum powder. Sue is standing beside Becky and I am sitting on the side of the bath. I ask Sue about the therapeutic value of the aroma of lily of the valley and she says she doesn't know what it is. I tell them both that I love the scent and that it also reminds me of my grandmother and the verse in the Bible referring to the Lord as 'the Lily of the valley, the bright and morning star.'

Becky says that she loves the scent also and that she has used it for forty years or so. She says her husband asked her recently what she wanted for a birthday and she replied that she would like some of her favourite perfume and he didn't know what it was. She begins to cry and says that it has been sitting on the shelf in front of him all that time and he didn't even know.

Becky says she has done everything for him and that she doesn't ask much in return. We are all quiet. Sue tells Becky how good it is that she is crying, because she hasn't been able to show her emotions. Becky is crying softly and begins to dress herself with some assistance from Sue. Sue mainly stands back a little and lets Becky do what she can for herself. Sue asks whether she would like to clean her teeth and Becky pulls the chair around and begins to take out her dentures and clean them with toothpaste. They are talking most of the time about Becky's need to cry and the ways in which the oils can help her to cope with the pain. They are calm and easy with one another. There is a sense of patience here.

It is time to go back to the bed. Becky stands up and leaves the bathroom with Sue walking beside her. I carry the dressing gown and walk behind them. Becky says she is exhausted. Sue suggests she could lie down on her bed if she likes. When they approach the bed, Sue puts Becky's toiletries away in the bedside locker and goes to make her a cup of tea. Sue knows that Becky takes milk and sugar in her tea. Becky settles on the bed and I tell her I'll come back to talk with her after her cup of tea and when she's had a rest.

Interpretations

Becky was feeling miserable with the pain of her broken rib, which was a consequence of osteoporosis, which in turn could be traced to a lack of oestrogen following an oophorectomy years ago. However, Becky's pain was not only physical; she was working through some long-standing pain about her relationship with her husband and with other people in her life, who had tended to take her for granted. Becky was ready for rebellion. She was ready to break out into a different lifestyle, in which she counted herself as important.

Becky said this to sum up her situation: 'You're born somebody's daughter, then you're somebody's wife, you're somebody's mother, somebody's grandmother. When is it going to be time for me?'

I accompanied Becky and Sue to the bathroom one morning, as Sue prepared an aromatherapy bath. Sue had taken time to get to know Becky and she encouraged the outpouring of tears, that were beginning to unleash Becky's sense of entrapment. I analysed the text relating to the interaction between Sue and Becky and eight main qualities and activities emerged, which were: appreciating skilful nursing care; expressing feelings; acknowledging the relevance of family affiliations; facilitating independence; facilitating changes; relating to the other's situation; enjoying a sense of humour; and preparing to go home.

Appreciating skilful nursing care. As a result of lack of oestrogen replacement after her internal reproductive organs were removed, Becky developed osteoporosis and, subsequently, a broken rib. She was also mentally depressed. Sue prepared an aromatherapy bath for Becky and assisted her to get into and out of it. For Becky the bath meant more than the bath itself; it also symbolised the way in which Sue was attempting to allow her to regain confidence in herself. Becky said:

> '*What I liked about the bath was it was hot. It took the pain away. It made me sleepy. I feel Sue's begun to give me a bit of confidence back. I don't really know. She makes me feel that I am going to get better. I can do things.*'

Sue explained the intentions and outcomes of the bath.

> 'So, in a sense I suppose, what I was doing with Becky this morning, was not a bath but a reaction to the aromatherapies, to see if, (a) we could use oils to help her, and (b) whether we could use some touch therapy with a massage later on. She has refused massages for two days and yet after the bath she said she would love to have a massage with oils, so it seems the bath was the mechanism to help her to have decreased pain, to relax, and to help her cry. She is now going to have some tactile therapy to help her cry some more and get all those negative feelings out she's got inside, that she has held inside for twenty-five years. So the bath was a medium to use other therapeutic agents. It worked out well. I think the other thing about today's bath is that she was very down beforehand. She said to me: "I can't get anything right." She was very negative about the bath, but afterwards she was very positive.'

Expressing feelings. During her stay in the PNU Becky released emotions, which had been stored up for at least twenty-five years. Becky was ambivalent about crying, because she was concerned about what other people might think of her. She appreciated the way Sue encouraged her to express her feelings.

> '*But people think that you're soft because you cry. I've got nobody to turn to. You've got to work yourself out...but Sue really is [helpful], when I cry she doesn't try and shut me up.*'

Becky expressed how she felt about her life circumstances.

'You're born somebody's daughter, then you're somebody's wife, you're somebody's mother, somebody's grandmother. When is it going to be time for me! I want to be just me! I've always done it [helped other people], so you just do it. Becky gets a bit tired. Never mind, I'll get there eventually.'

Sue expressed how she felt about the tears, which were flooding from Becky.

'But it's great, as she says, she hasn't cried for twenty-five years and she is entitled! I thought it was good. It was good that she came out of the bath and was relaxed and that she felt comfortable enough to cry, because she is a strong lady and so used to being very strong, that showing her weakness is a real no-no. So, for her it is terrific, because she did it in front of two people and felt good about doing it, in her nakedness of all things! She was sitting there starkers and crying. Now, if that isn't trust, I'd hate to think what would be. She was at her most vulnerable and she felt good about the two people she was with. If she wants to cry, let her!'

Acknowledging the relevance of family affiliations. Becky explained the influence her husband had in limiting her independence after her last operation.

'When somebody has been telling you that "You can't do that and you can't do this and you can't do something else!" You get to feel that you're no use at all to anybody...My husband says to me: "You can't do that, you can't do that!"...I know there's a lot of things that I can't do at the moment. I know that I'm back in here because I got stubborn and I asked him to put the washing on the line and he fell asleep in the chair and I got cross and I went out and did it myself and that's what started all this pain up again. But to be told you can't do it. At least give me the chance to try and then be able to say: "I can't do that—you'll have to do it." But he doesn't do that, he just says: "You can't do it," just because he won't do it."'

Becky expressed how it felt to be dependent on her husband's help.

'I've never depended on other people to do things for me, I've always done things for myself and for the family...I've always done everything for everybody else. I know that now. "Becky will do that!" Becky will look after him [her husband] and Becky has got to the stage where she's tired of looking after him. We talk about things to buy, and do things. But I'm the one that has to remember to pay the bills and remember to make sure that the money's in the bank. He doesn't know how to do it. He honestly doesn't know how to do it. But he doesn't want to learn now.'

Facilitating independence. Becky wanted to regain her independence and Sue helped her towards fulfilling her goal.

'I was beginning to think I was just useless. But Sue makes me feel I'm not that bad and I will get better, but it will take time. If I can control the pain. Sue said to me: "If you want me, ring [the buzzer]." When I've

wanted her I've rung and she came and she didn't insist that she help me and that's what I like. She didn't say: "Oh you can't do that. I've got to help you." She just let me go and therefore if I was looking as though I was going to get into trouble she'd help me, but she let me go and let me do it by myself and that's what I want to do. I didn't need to be babied. To be told: "Now be careful, don't do this and don't do that!" She just let me go. If I looked as if I was going to get into trouble, she got her hand ready. That's all I wanted. I don't want somebody there, saying: "Careful about this!" Even getting undressed and getting dressed, people said [that] to me.

Sue said: "Can you do that? Can you dress and undress yourself?" and I said: "Yes." I know I look awkward doing it, but I've worked it out how to do it without hurting myself. Sue just lets me go. When I want help she's there and so are the other girls [nurses], they're there. They'll help. I want to try and do things by myself and they just let me go and that's all I want and I feel that I'll get better quicker.'

Facilitating changes. Becky began to see alternatives for action when she returned home to her husband, and she accredited Sue with some praise for opening up her mind to the various choices. Becky said:

'If he [my husband] wants things done, he'll have to do them himself. I don't think he can do it, because he's there on his own most of the time. David [our son] comes over and looks after him at night and gets his meals, but he'll look after himself. Sue's made me see that. She's made me realise that I can do things, so I don't have to have somebody there to hold my hand. I don't need that. I just need help every now and again when I get stuck. When I get something caught or I can't get out, and that's what she does for me. She makes me feel useful. [Becky begins to cry]. Gee I'm an awful cry-baby aren't I? I'm just going to start saying: "No!" to people. I'll just say: "No, I haven't got time for that. I've got something else to do!" [I'll] go back to bowls. I'll go on the trips with them. If he don't want to go, he can stay home.'

Relating to the other's situation. Sue related to Becky's distress and described the sort of nursing care that she thought Becky needed to help her through her dilemma.

'I think her first need is talking, just to have a listening ear and to have someone tell her that she can let loose to cry, scream, shout. If we had a shouting room it would be ideal for her. Her emotional needs are first, then her physical and she obviously needs pain control and she needs to see why she is nauseated and vomiting.'

Enjoying a sense of humour. Sue joked with Becky when she was waiting for Becky to get herself out of the bath, about the way Becky had devised for herself, and Sue was thrilled when Becky 'cracked a joke,' when she was getting dressed after her bath. Sue said:

'At the end of it [her bath], she actually cracked a joke, which I picked up on. It was the first time I heard her crack a joke, when I said to her: "Twenty-five years ago the doctors stuffed up your hormones." After she cried, she said: "Twenty-five years ago I wouldn't know what was going on!" She actually gave me a wicked grin on the side. Now, that was an incredible reaction. It was the first time I've seen that lady give any type of spontaneous smile or any type of warmth, because she is just so down. It was great that the wickedness came out of her, because it was a wicked statement. She was having a go at the system. She wasn't crying at it and she wasn't angry at it, but she was saying: "Well, I wouldn't know what to do either."'

Preparing to go home. Becky was destined to go home, when she was able to walk freely. Sue realised that Becky also needed some coping strategies to assist her with her home situation.

> 'She is supposed to stay in until she can fully mobilise, but because her husband wants one hundred percent attendance, I think with this lady in particular, it will be when she is ready to go home. I can't see anyone pushing her out the door, because they [the doctors] know it [her condition] is iatrogenic [caused by medical treatment] and the nursing staff won't suggest it [going home] until she is walking around reasonably comfortably and is able to cope with her husband. She needs coping mechanisms. As she talks more people will be able to say: "Well, have you tried this or have you tried that?" She has to relearn her patterns…She has spent so much time talking about it [her problem] over the last few days that it is starting to fall into place. She knows she has to look after herself.'

Conclusions

Sue knew Becky from the time she has been admitted. Becky shared many details of her home life with Sue, who came to know what was important for Becky at that time in her life. Becky was in pain and she was depressed. Her problems stemmed in part from lack of oestrogen replacement after some gynaecological surgery years ago and from the patterns she had set up in her own life.

Becky expressed the need to be as independent as she could be and she did not want to be constrained by other people's impressions of what she was capable of doing. Sue offered to help Becky as she needed it, but waited to be asked. She was there for Becky, not hovering, but back out of the way, so that Becky felt she had space to be herself and to do things her way, in her time.

Becky was tied to fulfilling other people's needs, especially her husband's, rather than living her own life as she chose. Becky started to deal with the pent up emotions of twenty-five years and it involved much crying and talking. Sue accepted and encouraged her tears and expression of feelings. Even though Becky was weighed down with pain and depression, she was starting to see that she could make other choices for herself. Becky was appreciative of the ways in which Sue helped her to find what her choices might be.

Sue accepted Becky's tears and allowed her to do what she wanted to do for herself. Sue was sensitive to Becky's needs and she provided acceptance, company, humour and the offer of support to Becky. Sue knew that Becky was the only person who could make changes in her own life patterns and she was with her to help her discover those choices.

Introducing Naomi

Naomi was born on 18 May 1911. She lives with her daughter and son-in-law in their two storey house. Naomi has three other daughters, all of whom are happy to have their mother live with them after her operation. She has essential hypertension and systemic lupus erythematosis, but an occlusion of her right superior femoral artery and the resultant gangrene in her first and third toes has necessitated a below knee amputation She is rehabilitating presently in the PNU and will be transferring to another centre soon, to be assisted with prosthesis fitting and mobilisation.

Sue and Naomi: a story about accepting body image changes

It is about 9.30 a.m. Naomi is sitting in her wheelchair in her space in a four bed ward. She has her right leg stretched out horizontally at waist level on a splint, which is at the front of the chair. Her right leg terminates below the knee in a cupped shape, which is sporting a healing wound line, now devoid of sutures. It is a small leg, proportionate to the stature of the woman. Her left leg is bent at the knee and her intact foot rests on the foot plate of the wheelchair. She is bright-eyed and alert.

Her mind is keen; this I know personally, because we have talked before. On those occasions she told me about her childhood, how she was adopted as a baby, and how she later found out the identity of her mother, and got to know an old aunt, who is a Catholic Sister. She told me about her name, how she is christened one name and is known by another. She told me about her grandson, and the tragedy he has experienced in his life. We have talked before and she remembers my name.

Naomi's chair is between her bed and the window. The curtains are open and the morning sun is streaming in. I am sitting on the bed, facing Naomi. As I sit beside Naomi, Sue approaches us both, smiling. She points to Naomi's left leg. 'Did she tell you about that?' she asks, and quickly continues to explain that she is referring specifically to a reddened area, which became apparent just above Naomi's left knee yesterday.

Sue says she thinks the reddened area was due to the bandaging and that she was concerned that it may have caused the skin to breakdown. Sue says that the bandage was too tight, but Naomi didn't want to 'wake' the night staff. Naomi quickly agrees, saying that she does not want to be a nuisance. Sue assures her that it is OK to speak up when she needs something. As she speaks, Sue is bent down over the wheelchair, touching the area and making gentle, circular rubbing movements over the bony prominence.

Sue's eyes move between Naomi and myself. Naomi is listening to and endorsing Sue's comments. Naomi says that the red spot is hardly noticeable today. The attention then shifts to a skin flap at the side of the stump. Naomi asks whether this will be OK. Sue assures her that the prosthesis will fit well and that the small flap will not hinder her rehabilitation.

They talk about the impending transfer to a rehabilitation centre. It will be here that Naomi will learn to walk with the help of a prosthesis. Sue talks with her about what it will mean, and answers questions Naomi raises, such as whether she will be able to get herself into bed. The interaction is unhurried and centred on Naomi. The conversation is over in about five minutes. Naomi is waiting to go for her shower. We leave her sitting beside her bed.

Interpretations

Naomi was recovering in the PNU, following an amputation of her left leg. To the casual visitor to the nursing unit, Naomi appeared to have fared well after the operation, however, Sue had been with her and she knew that Naomi had many fears and concerns. Sue waited until Naomi was ready, and she watched Naomi, as she finally accepted the stump as part of herself. In the interaction in which I was present, Sue discussed a reddened area on Naomi's stump with her and made the observation that the flap was looking ready for the prosthesis.

Five main qualities and activities emerged from an analysis of the text relating to the interaction between Sue and Naomi, and these were: relating to the nurse as person; giving confidence; relating to the other's situation; facilitating acceptance of body image changes; and acknowledging the importance of company and talking

Relating to the nurse as person. Naomi explained how she regarded Sue.

> 'Well, she seems to be such a normal sort of, she's a nurse, but as well as being a nurse, she's a friendly sort of person, who gives you confidence, I think. That makes a big difference doesn't it, you don't look at her as a clinical sort of figure altogether, she's a friend as well. It's hard to explain. Well, when I say normal, to me normal is to be friendly and helpful, as well as being that trained person, who knows what it's all about anyway, but you feel that you can talk to her as a friend. Not to be afraid to ask questions, whether it be foolish or not. Because she treats very sensibly and in a friendly manner. I just can't explain it…I don't have to be afraid of her training and because she knows so much about this and that, that I'm scared of asking her something. I don't feel like that at all. I feel I can ask her anything, sensible or not.'

Giving confidence. Naomi was appreciative of the ways in which Sue and some other nurses gave her confidence.

> 'Well she [Sue] was really wonderful I thought. She gives you great confidence. That's my opinion of her…Also, Janice has been wonderful too. She gave me great confidence when I was having a blood transfusion, which I've never had before in my life, and I was petrified. I said to her: 'I'm scared,' and she said, (who else was there, was it Hazel?), they'd play a tape for me, a relaxing tape. I hate to see blood in bottles and after about a quarter of an hour I was so relaxed with them being around me and being so calm and confident and helping me in that respect, that I began to relax with them too, apart from the tape, it was very good. And also because they [the doctors] have a lot of trouble getting the veins and while they're doing that, they [the nurses] are reassuring me that "It's not going to be long now, a vein is going to pop up that's not a slippery one" and we began to laugh about it instead of being tense. They've been really wonderful.'

Relating to the other's situation. Sue knew Naomi well enough to know that she was an anxious person. Sue related to how Naomi might be feeling about the reddened area on her stump and her forthcoming transfer to the rehabilitation centre.

> 'We were looking at it [the spot on Naomi's stump] this morning just to see how red it was, how sore it was and how she generally felt about it, because she's a very anxious lady, and going out to [the rehabilitation centre] alone was very frightening for her. She didn't need that added worry of what the redness might mean…I think the thing that was in the back of my mind the whole time, was the fact that she was so anxious about going to the centre. She fell once and she just chastised herself the whole time for being stupid, for damaging the stump. She was just so hysterical. And it was just purely a thing where she lent out of her chair and the chair gave way, so she wasn't aware of it, and from that we've learnt she was a lady, who was very very scared obviously after the amputation

that something was going to go wrong, that a complication could set in and things would go bad for her.'

Facilitating acceptance of body image changes. Sue helped Naomi to accept her stump as part of her, but in Naomi's own time and way. Sue explained:

'We put it to her yesterday to have a look at the bottom part of her stump. I said I'd go away and get a mirror and she said: "No, I've got one," in other words to me it was, "I'll do it when I'm ready." Then she actually [her daughter was there] and she was very hesitant, she brought it over very slowly. I think what it was that she could whip it away if she didn't like what she saw. But then when she saw it, she spent a good five minutes going from all angles and going: "Isn't that wonderful, that's fantastic!" So we went through again what they'd done at the operation, and this time it actually sank in, because she could see it. But she wasn't ready until that time. That was three weeks post-op. She wasn't ready until then to have a look. That was her timing and that's when she did it. That was the thing about her, her timing. I can remember the first day she did it [massaged her stump], she was so tentative. She was so frightened of touching it. So I just took her through a few massage techniques, and said: "It's really nice if you just give it a rub like this. If you do this, if you do that, you'll feel really good." You could see her through the day, the circles were getting bigger and bigger and more firmer and the hands and the stump were an item. It wasn't a stump, that she was kind of barely touching. It was beautiful the way you could see it happening.'

Acknowledging the importance of company and talking. Sue recognised Naomi's need for reassurance, especially with the impending transfer out of the PNU.

'She needed a lot of staff contact this morning, and she needed as much confidence as she could get, before she actually made that move to go out to the centre. So, just the past experiences of working with her in the last couple of weeks, today you knew you had to spend that little bit of extra time with her to get her confidence right up, [to help her] feel really good in herself, [to] feel that things are going well, [and to] explain what was happening out at the centre, what they will do with her, and allow her to talk about any other fears…A strange environment is going to be hard for her, and I think that was in the back of my mind as soon as I came on duty, the fact that she'd need that time.'

Conclusions

Naomi was a woman who had an interesting life and she shared her family events with people who would listen. She spoke calmly of how she was adopted and how she contacted her natural mother's aunt, who was a Catholic nun. She recalled her grandson's tragedy and although the story was very sad, she managed to tell it through without tears. This bright woman was articulate. She expressed her external life events, however, she was not adept at expressing her inner feelings.

Naomi seemed to be managing her recent leg amputation well. To the casual outsider, she seemed 'together' and in total control of her situation. However, Sue knew a different Naomi. Sue knew the Naomi who chastised herself so severely for falling out of her wheelchair, the Naomi who didn't want to bother the night nurses when her bandage was tight, the Naomi who had only just recently accepted the sight and touch of her amputated leg.

Sue knew Naomi after three weeks in the unit, during which time Sue had seen Naomi get accustomed to, and begin to own and care for, her own stump. Sue knew that Naomi was actually an anxious woman; she had deduced this after being with Naomi for a large part of the last three weeks, talking with her and caring for her.

Sue knew that the latest issue of the reddened spot on Naomi's stump was potentially problematic for Naomi, in that she was soon to be transferred to a strange, new centre and the apprehension of it, together with the worry of her stump, might have been overwhelming for her. So, Sue spent time with Naomi, talking about the disappearance of the reddened area and Naomi's imminent transfer. She knew Naomi and cared about how she was feeling about her world at that time.

Naomi appreciated the way that Sue was 'normal,' that is, how she knew so much professionally, yet she could still be friendly and make Naomi feel at ease. Naomi was willing to say anything and ask anything, because she knew that Sue would not think it was trivial in any way. To Naomi, Sue was a professional, who could be knowledgeable, but also friendly, helpful and accepting of her, in all her humanness.

Introducing Patrick

Patrick was born on 31 May 1956. He lives alone, is divorced, and has a history of family problems. He was admitted to hospital through the Accident and Emergency section, having ingested seventy milligrams of diazepam (Valium), two flagons of sherry and possibly he had also taken smack (Heroin). Patrick was transferred to the PNU the next day for detoxification. He has been admitted to the PNU three times before for similar reasons. He is to be discharged from the unit tomorrow, without diazepam.

Sue and Patrick: a story about addiction

Sue and I walk to Patrick together. He is at the end of a corridor opening out to the sunroom, at the front of the building. The corridor is skirted by beds, one after the other in line. Patrick's area is on the left, on the way to the sunroom. The window at the side of his area is admitting brilliant sunshine. There is a smell of the aftershave lotion Old Spice in the air.

A blue cap is hanging from the sky hook above the centre of Patrick's bed. The bed is clean and without a wrinkle. Patrick's bedside locker has a blue tray cover on top and on it are arranged various toiletries and personal belongings in neat order. I comment: 'That looks neat,' looking at Patrick. Sue says: 'That's part of your problem isn't it Patrick. You are obsessive-compulsive.' Patrick doesn't answer, but walks around to take his watch off the locker. 'That's another thing,' she says, 'he also paces.'

There is an awkward time, as we decide what will happen. Sue suggests that we go to Patrick's favourite place, to which Patrick responds: 'What do you need sunshine for?' So, we settle on the window side of Patrick's bed. Sue and Patrick sit in chairs facing each other at a distance. Sue is up one end, Patrick up the other and I am sitting on the bed in the centre. It looks and it feels awkward to me. I say that I would like to move, because I don't want to intervene in their discussion and I move to the other side of the bed. Sue changes her position, moving her chair closer to Patrick.

Sue introduces the aim of the talk, that is, to talk about the ways in which this impending discharge from hospital will differ from the other times. Patrick is hesitant to speak at first. Behind us we hear the tune: 'Carol County Accident.' Sue says that she brought the music in for Max and that particular song is her favourite. The noise of the traffic outside on the busy street is coming loudly through the window. Patrick is sitting with his arms crossed, leaning into the oxygen apparatus on the wall.

It is a stilted and self-conscious interaction, made different from usual, I imagine, by my presence as a participant observer. On several occasions Sue tries to assure Patrick that it is OK to talk. She tells Patrick not to worry about me, saying: 'She's a good woman. You can trust Bev.' I am very aware of the effect I am having on this interaction, although I am for all the world trying to pretend I'm invisible.

At one stage they are discussing a previous admission, when he didn't want the PNU staff to know he was in hospital. Sue says: 'If you come in again, I will never speak to you again.' He doesn't look alarmed by this statement. I wonder about this statement. A voice calls to Sue to tell her someone is here to see her. 'Can you tell him to wait a minute?' she asks. Sue and Patrick continue the interaction, but they both seem uncomfortable. Patrick closes the window and comments on 'that awful music in the background,' knowing that Sue has just expressed previously a love of country music. It is nearly midday. Sue says: 'I'll be back to see you about 3.30 p.m. I'm going on days off and I won't see you when you go. You make sure you're here!' I'm pleased that she will be seeing him again, because I feel that they will have a chance to really talk then.

Interpretations

Using the method discussed previously in Chapter 2, I located eight main qualities and activities from my analysis of the text relating to the interaction between Sue and Patrick, which appeared to illuminate the phenomenon of ordinariness in nursing. The qualities and activities were: expressing feelings; enjoying a sense of humour; relating to the genuineness in people; expressing affection and liking; talking straight; feeling comfortable; relating to the other's situation and relating to the patient as person.

Expressing feelings. The interaction between Patrick and Sue was stilted and unlike their usual dialogue. Patrick expressed how he felt about the interaction.

> 'I was a little bit nervous. I guess because of the third party [the researcher], nothing against the third party. It was OK. I guess I wasn't more sort of spontaneous and little more jovial and spoke off my own bat. I was pre-occupied with the fact that I know my discharge date and I've got this accommodation thing and stuff like that.'

Sue also expressed her feelings in relation to the interaction. Sue said:

> 'This morning was a disaster from my point of view. Patrick and I were both incredibly stilted. We just didn't interact at all. It was very embarrassing. I could feel myself going red while I was talking to him. I was trying every body position in the world to relax. I don't think I stopped moving the whole time! Didn't you notice it?
> I was watching Patrick and he had the closed-off body language. Then I saw his feet moving and I thought "He's either got haemorrhoids or he's got the same problem I've got!" Then he closed the window and I thought "Oh God this is awful!" It's stuff that we have talked about time and time again. It's just amazing. I think that when we talk, it's very private.

I said: "Let's go out to your favourite spot" and he said: "Why?" and I thought "This is going to be a failure" instantly. He was staying in a room where people could hear him and he thought "Sue's not going to ask me anything that could be embarrassing, because we've got all these people around us." He was wrong, but still, that's what he was thinking. I'd say this morning from the last x-amount of times that I've been with Patrick, today would have to be a wipe-out. I don't think anything was achieved. We both knew that we were talking for the sake of talking.'

Patrick expressed how he felt about being readmitted to the PNU

'Oh because the last time I left, the impression they [the nurses] got, or I believed they had anyway, is that this time I'd make a good go of it and I didn't. I couldn't face sort of being seen again. "Here he is. He's stuffed up again. He's done it again!"'

Sue described how Patrick expressed his feelings, when he had to be readmitted to the PNU

'Like I said, it's the fourth time around and I just find it really sad that he said: "Don't let the unit know." The whole time I brought him over here, he said: "Oh they're going to look down at me." I said: "No, no one's going to look down at you." He said: "I'm so ashamed." He was crying. "I'm so ashamed, so ashamed."

Enjoying a sense of humour. Patrick and Sue knew each other well enough to joke about the most serious of subjects. Sue told him that if he came back, she would never speak to him again. Patrick gave a retort that only Sue and he could appreciate.

'Oh it's just a bit of a joke. If I come back on a slab, meaning if I come back dead. She said that to me a couple of days ago and I said: "I won't be talking to anyone!"'

Relating to the genuineness in people. Patrick claimed that he could sense genuineness in people. He found genuineness in Sue. Patrick said of Sue:

'I find her very easy to talk to. If I had a problem or whatever or a query, she would be the one I would see...I believe she's genuine...well I've always considered myself a good judge of character. It's a feeling I get, that there is genuine concern.'

Patrick compared Sue's genuineness to some of the other people with whom he interacted over various stays in hospital.

'It's not like some of the nurses. Some of the other nurses, you can tell that when you speak to them, that they're not really, they're hearing you, but they're not really listening to you. When you've finished, basically it's going in one ear and out the other. They don't really give a damn.

Like there are nurses and there are nurses, and there are doctors and there are doctors. Like I say, there's the ones that it goes in one ear and out the other, don't really care. Like I was talking to a particular nurse the other night, to me she's that sort of person, I don't like her. If I'm walking down the corridor and she's walking the other way, I'll just look straight ahead. I won't acknowledge her or anything like that, because I know that she doesn't give a damn. In other words, you get the odd nurse that will come up and she'll talk with you. She's genuine. I'm not saying this is the only ward in the hospital that's got good nurses, but I think that on this ward, I find that you can more or less mix in with them.'

Expressing affection and liking. Patrick appreciated Sue's friendliness. He said:

(Very long pause) 'I guess there's been more than one occasion. She'll always say 'Hello!' to you. She treats you like a friend. It's hard to explain.'

Talking straight. Patrick and Sue were accustomed to speaking very clearly and frankly to one another. Patrick appreciated Sue's forthrightness. He explained it in this way:

'If I sort of had time to really think about it, I could come up with a specific thing, but I know that she's no good as a 'yes man.' If the doctor or what not said, "This guy should go, I think it's time he left," and she believed he wasn't ready to go, well she'd say so.'

Sue often talked straight to Patrick and she explained why she did this.

'I can see the potential and there's not a damn thing I can do about it, because it's all up to him, except to be there as a sounding board, not really a sounding board, because I attack him, but at least with the attacks I get answers back again at me. I think it's because of that relationship that has formed especially over the last two admissions.'

Sue spoke frankly to her colleagues in relation to Patrick's care. He had been admitted to another ward and did not want the nursing staff at the PNU to know. Sue explained:

'This admission, he'd been left for over 24 hours without Valium. They didn't do anything until I went up [to another ward] and saw him, and he was nearly fitting. Then I went up to the ward and said: "Do you realise this guy's about to fit?" Action stations! So, I'd rather know that he was in [hospital], and know that he's alright, and that he had some medication, than to know that he was suffering up in a ward somewhere, and no one was giving a brass razoo about him. He was just Patrick. Oh in again, OD (overdose), big deal!'

However, most of Sue's straight talking was reserved for Patrick, when she felt he needed it.

'Patrick said to me one day that he didn't want to go to the local psychiatric centre, because of the stigma. I said: "What bloody stigma. Don't talk to me about stigmas! Look what has happened to you [being ignored by health carers], because of a stigma! So don't you talk to me about stigmas. You've had enough of it, so don't you start doing it now!"'

On another occasion, Sue said:

'The second admission he was scoring [picking up drugs] out the front, so the third admission I said to him: "You lie to me and I'll bash your head in!" So he was fine, he was straight [not deceitful] the whole time. I said: "If you have it [drugs], fine, I don't care, just don't treat me like an idiot!"'

Sue explained why she used such straight language with Patrick.

'I think that's probably the main thing is, that you tend to, you talk to them like you talk to a friend, who had a habit. I mean most of us know someone, who has got some type of problem somewhere along the line. Even if they don't even admit to it half the time. It could be husbands, it could be children, it could be anything.'

Feeling comfortable. Patrick described the degree of comfortableness he felt with being in hospital and interacting with some people.

'Over the years, I've been in this hospital a fair few times. The staff, you can't beat these people. Well, with the exception of one or two, I feel comfortable. A hospital is for people, who are sick. When you're sick in hospital, you generally wear pyjamas. Even though, for me, hospital and pyjamas go together, you still seem to stand out, you know what I mean. Whereas in this unit, you can get around in your civvies, you don't seem to stick out like a sore thumb. Even though, like this morning, I was last in having a shower and I was still getting around in my pyjamas, about 10 o'clock. And I was walking round in my pyjamas amongst all these people walking around in clothes and I felt comfortable. I didn't feel as though I stuck out like a sore thumb.

Just even going outside and sitting and having a cigarette and that, was because the staff and that made me feel good. I felt good, the fact that I had pyjamas on, it didn't worry me going outside to have a cigarette, and cars driving past and people walking in and out, it didn't worry me. When I feel comfortable I act naturally.'

Relating to the other's situation. Sue and Patrick's to each other's situation over a history of four admissions. Sue explained:

'As you know, it's his fourth time round. I didn't get to know him very well on his first visit, he was only in for a couple of days. But I started to get to know him better on the second. I think it was probably the third admission we had Patrick in that I think the rapport started. I remember I was massaging his back and that's the only time I've ever massaged him and had any type of hands-on contact, because he maintains that body distance. He turned around and said: "I was just about to ask you a private question," and I said: "That's alright. No problems. What is it?" He said: "Why aren't you married?" I said: "Well people keep falling off their white horses and dropping their shining armour, and it just hasn't worked out!"'

Then we talked about his marriage, which has been an incredibly painful experience for him. He was married to a psychiatric-trained Registered Nurse. I think it was through that massage a lot of barriers were broken and since that time we've gone forward.

That's where the trigger seems to hit with me. It was from that massage, because it was the first time that he actually had a massage. Before that he wouldn't use the oils. He wouldn't have anything to do with them. I still think at this stage we're on a no-win situation and I've told Patrick that I think he will bounce back in again.'

Sue and Patrick shared their self-disclosures. Sue said:

'It's such a personal and such an emotive issue when you're talking about growth, and patient's addiction and stuff like that. With Patrick being used to me opening up about my life and then he opens up about his life, and therefore it's an emotive issue on both sides.'

Sue explained how she came to relate to Patrick's situation.

'I think my personal feelings about Patrick have been very much influenced by reading his history. He comes into Accident and Emergency, he's given Narcane [an antidote for narcotic overdose] and is escorted to the front door. Quote, unquote "This patient is not to be admitted."'

I see this guy who's so clean and his clothes are washed every day. In the history, and I'm reading it, I was nearly in tears. Patrick and I sat there one night and we went through his history and it was OD'd [overdosed] this, that and the other; and all the agents he'd been through. I thought, "Here's this really clean guy." He is obsessive and compulsive. I'm convinced of it, with his clothes and everything. He used to be in the army, so it could be a backdrop to that. This guy rolling in urine, coming into Accident and Emergency, spaced-out, vomiting all over everything.'

Sue imagined how Patrick might have felt about his emergency admissions.

'It must be so degrading to think back on that's the way he came in. I read it out (not that part). I said to him: "Check this out" and we went through his admission and the way he'd been shown to the front door and we went through things and I said: "Look, this time, you're not going to make it. You were almost dead there. Look at how close you were. Look at your statistics and stuff like that and your obs; you were nearly dead. Now what's going to happen next time? You are going to end up on that slab."

I don't know. I have this awful feeling that that's what's going to happen.'

In relating to his situation, Sue concluded that Patrick was worth the attention paid to him and questioned the tendency of health professionals to treat him as 'nuisance value'.

'Just reading through his history, I think "Well he's had an abused childhood and he started on the stuff, and his marriage broke up, and he's been through a lot." OK, some people cope, some people don't. With him, I find that he is a very closed person, who can't...If he could get a group of people around him that he could talk to, I think he'd be alright. But his family have pretty well disowned him now. So I think it's up to the nursing profession to at least do something while he's here and not just say: "Oh God he's back again!" I find that if you read his history, you'd just say: "Did we [nurses and doctors] really do that? Did we throw someone out on the street again?" Then you get into those arguments of whether you have a de-tox [someone who is undergoing detoxification from drugs] taking up the bed of someone critical.'

Relating to the patient as person. Sue related to Patrick as a person. She imagined how she might feel if he 'came in on a slab' (dead) sometime.

'But, to me, a person's a person. Some people would say I'm overly attached to Patrick in a sense. I think the fact of having got so close to him over the last four admissions, and that I do like him as a patient and a person as well. So, it would be the same as having someone who I work with basically, that's a work acquaintance, the same thing happening to them. Patrick's someone who's been in so often, that I've got to know him as well as I've got to know the people who I work with. I don't socialise with Patrick, but within a working relationship you're close to people here and you care about what happens to them. And I mean you've [the researcher has] just joined the team in a sense, but if something happened to you, we'd all be cot-cases, because we've got to know you and like you and that's the same way I react to Patrick, that I've got to know him in that working relationship, so if he came in, to me it would be such an incredible waste for someone.'

Sue knew Patrick as a person with potential.

'I've seen him work with the oldies [older people]. I've seen him feed them and get cross with nursing staff, who haven't come to the room to help the person in time and they've got themselves in a mess. He's walked debilitated patients to the toilet, so they wouldn't wee themselves. He loves being involved. That's the really sad part. He could be a wardsman or something like that, where he could be involved. Even though he claims not to like the hospital environment, it's a very important part to him.'

Conclusions

Sue and Patrick had built a trusting relationship. It came as no surprise to the researcher, that the planned interaction was stilted, because it lacked the essential ingredients of their relationship: the two of them, sitting quietly together, in privacy. When he was alone with Sue, he opened himself up to her, just as she shared some of herself with him. He knew that Sue was genuine in her concern for him.

Patrick appreciated Sue's genuineness. She treated him like a friend. He felt he could tell the difference between nurses who were genuine and those who 'didn't give a damn.' The degree of genuineness was related to the concern he felt they had for him, in being prepared to talk with him in an attentive, caring way.

Patrick became accustomed to hospital life, over successive admissions, but he still felt some discomfort about conforming to the patient role, especially in relation to wearing pyjamas during the day. Patrick said that when he felt comfortable, he acted naturally. The nurses and the unit made him feel comfortable, and because he was comfortable in the PNU he felt natural. The comfortableness had the potential to make him feel more natural, so he was more likely to be able to be honest with himself about his dependency or whatever else he was looking at in his life.

Sue talked straight to him and he responded in kind. In response to her comment: 'If you come back again, I won't talk to you,' he quipped that if he was brought in on a slab, he wouldn't be able to talk with her. Their humour was of a special kind; it was possible because they knew they could 'shoot from the hip' and say what it was they wanted to say to each other, albeit through the medium of humour sometimes.

Patrick was embarrassed about his recurrent trips to Accident and Emergency and to the PNU. He felt that people would think he was a 'no-hoper.' Sue wanted him to let her know if and when he came into hospital again, because she felt he could be in the unit, where people cared about him as a person and didn't treat him like 'just another OD'.

Sue saw Patrick's potential and she felt sorry when other people treated him like he was a hopeless case. She saw a clean, tidy man and felt sad for the degradation Patrick must have being in a complete mess, when he was admitted through Accident and Emergency. Together they went through the accounts of some of his admissions and they visited 'the bottom line,' that one day the treatment would not be successful and he would die from an overdose. Sue shared his stories and sensed some of his pain, but she felt he was in a 'no-win situation.'

Sue was a straight-talker where Patrick was concerned. She gave him her perception of things in no uncertain way; she did this because it caused a response in him and they could get their meanings clear. She talked to him clearly, because this was how she would talk to a friend, who had a habit.

Sue and Patrick enjoyed a rapport, which was born out of trusting closeness. Sue examined her own beliefs about closeness to patients and affirmed that it was OK. She cared about Patrick, but she was careful to point out that he had no obligation to her. If he died one day from an overdose, she acknowledged that that would be his choice and he would not have failed her personally. Sue will grieve for Patrick if he dies, just like she will for any other friend.

PART 3

Meanings

9. Ordinariness in nursing

The stories that have been related and interpreted in Chapters 3 to 8, are of everyday interactions that occurred between nurses and patients in the course of their daily existence in a nursing unit. These stories, and more, recounted in the thesis (Taylor 1991a), were the source of understanding ordinariness in nursing. The answers about what ordinariness in nursing might be, and the effects it might have, were hidden away within the language of the people involved in the research. It was my task to use a method that would unleash the meaning from the language and put it into some sort of order that was easy to assimilate, thus making its insights clear to myself, and to other readers of the research. In this part of the book I will describe ordinariness in nursing as it emerges from the stories represented in the whole thesis document and not only from the stories selected in this book. In this chapter you will notice the names of other characters in stories not told previously in this book. I have included other participants to give wider representation of how I came to interpret the phenomenon of ordinariness.

Qualitative research generates a great deal of information, because transcribed conversations tend to run into high multiple pages of written words. It is the responsibility of any researcher doing interpretive work to sift through the gathered information very carefully, so that the essence of its meaning can be salvaged. Other details, which appear to have no contextual bearing on the main intentions of the research, are put to one side. The salvaging of qualitative information is reminiscent of searching for gemstones of a certain type; some gems are of the desired type, others are precious but they are not the type being sought, and some of the other stones are clearly pieces of gravel stones and grit. All of the precious gems, and even the gravel, is stored separately for a time, in case it is needed at some time in the future, as an inspiration for other research questions.

After I had worked steadfastly through the phenomenological method I had devised for the research, I discovered that the ontological nature of the gems of the phenomenon of ordinariness, were within what I termed the aspects of the phenomenon. The aspects were those parts of the participants' dialogue that indicated the nature of the phenomenon, and these were made manifest to me when I used a hermeneutical form of enquiry into the transcribed text of all of the participants.

The language used by the people in the research not only illuminated the nature of the phenomenon, but it also shed some light on some of their own 'There-Being' as human beings, because, as they spoke their understandings about being together as patients and nurses, they spoke what they know about what it means to be humans interacting with other humans.

In line with Heidegger's reasoning about Being-in-the-world, the participants could not help but give me some clues as to the nature of Being, when they spoke of their everyday experiences, because they related their lived existence as people who have some understanding about the nature of existence itself. The people in the research embodied the phenomenon, and it was my task to listen to them speak their understandings of nursing, as they gained them in the temporo-spatial context of the nursing unit. As human beings living together relatively continuously in a world set apart for health care, patients and nurses were the ideal ones to speak of nursing and of their lived experience of the nursing unit. They spoke as individuals, yet their language conveyed representations of their intersubjective experiences of being together, as they made sense of their respective circumstances, as they unfolded within the nursing unit.

The nurses and patients were not people who were caught up in a time warp in the nursing unit. They had also lived within their respective private and public worlds at home, where they existed as 'non-patients' and 'non-nurses' and these home realities were connected inextricably to them. Thus, their own personal identities with other people and things in their lives, which were not connected directly to the nursing unit, were drawn with them into their experience of the unit, when they were there as patients and nurses. The multiplicities of their lived experiences outside the nursing unit were connected to them through past experiences, present perceptions, and future hopes; therefore, their Being-in-the-world applied to their perceptions of who they were as humans, and also of their relationships with other people and things in their lives, all of which they brought, in varying degrees, into their interpersonal encounters in the nursing unit.

The nurses and patients were people, first and foremost, and the nature of their humanness pervaded all that they were and did within the nursing unit. Therefore, when I explored the phenomenon, I also explored the humanness of these people, and this was accessed through their language, because it expressed their own existence as people; that is, their language expressed their understandings of their 'There-Being.'

As I have explained in Chapter 2, it is the prime intention of any phenomenological method to find the nature of 'the thing itself', and that is why I went into the nursing unit as a participant-observer and encouraged some nurses and patients there to share with me their understandings of their world. At this point of the analysis and interpretation of the research, I realised that I had only come part of the way towards uncovering the 'Dasein' or 'There-Being' of ordinariness, because even after naming and describing the aspects of the phenomenon, its ontological nature still remained somewhat hidden from me, along with any attempt that I might make to explicate of the nature of Being itself. If the research was to be phenomenological in the sense of it seeking to explicate Being, I had to go beyond the aspects of the phenomenon to what I have named its actualities. In this chapter, I will describe the aspects of the phenomenon before I explain how I went into the innermost areas of ordinariness, to gain some insights into how it reflected the nature of human existence itself.

The nature of the ordinariness: its aspects and the actualities

The nature of ordinariness in nursing reflected of the nature of some human beings who, at the time and for some time into their future, found themselves within the context of a health care institution. Whether they were living the experience of the nursing unit as nurses or patients, was to some extent irrelevant; they were humans within a relatively strange context, making sense of their experiences by whatever human means they had available to them.

Aspects of ordinariness

After I used an hermeneutical process in which the impressions of all of the nurse-patient interactions were merged and interpreted, I found that eight major aspects emerged as common to all the stories. I will address the aspects in alphabetical order in this chapter. There is no prioritisation of any of the aspects; none is greater or lesser that the other, because all of them shed some light on the nature of ordinariness in nursing. Each of the aspects has subsets, or qualities and activities, that make up its identity. The qualities and activities will be exemplified one by one, by presenting dialogue from the text. Some of the dialogue is drawn from stories of nurse-patient interactions not dealt with in this book. The full account of these stories can be found in my PhD thesis (Taylor 1991a).

The eight major aspects are: facilitation, fair play, familiarity, family, favouring, feelings, fun, and friendship.

Facilitation

Facilitation refers to the enabling qualities and activities of both nurses and patients, whereby certain challenges being experienced by one person are made easier to face by the other person. Some qualities and activities of facilitation include: appreciating skilful nursing care; appreciating help; facilitating independence; facilitating learning; facilitating coping; facilitating comfort; facilitating acceptance of body image changes; facilitating changes; calming fears; building trust; giving confidence; and allowing the experience to unfold.

Appreciating skilful nursing care. The nurses in the research were qualified nurses, registered to practice as competent practitioners. Without exception, their professional knowledge and skills were used daily in their interactions with patients, and this was borne out by the patients' impressions of their nursing care. The nurses were able to work skilfully, informed by the ever growing knowledge base of their professional education and their clinical experiences. The way in which the skilful nursing care was given was part of the nurses' Being-in-the-world of the PNU with patients; tasks and people were combined into a synchrony of seemingly effortless actions, which flowed according to the needs of each particular situation.

Donald expressed his appreciation of skilful work succinctly, when he said of Andrew:

> 'Well, he was always very conscientious in his work, he did his job very well...and we got along well together...[during the dressing of the wound] we'd talk about football, Andrew was [a supporter of] Essendon and I was [a supporter of] Collingwood and we used to throw a lot of rubbish at one another.'

Appreciating help. The patients required varying degrees of help from the nurses. Some of the patients were willing to express their need for help, others were hesitant to request help, while others relied entirely on the nurses to be in tune to any help they needed. Appreciating help was reciprocated by the nurses, who appreciated help from the patients in planning daily activities, that could best cater for their respective needs.

The reciprocity of appreciating help was exemplified nicely by the team work between Elizabeth and Coralina, who sat down together and worked out how they would go about helping Coralina. Elizabeth described how it happened for them both:

> 'Coralina gave me a big cuddle when she saw me and I said: "How difficult it must be for you to be in this situation" and she was a bit teary and she gave me a cuddle, and said: "Yeah." I said: "I'm sure we can work out a way that we could do it better than this." So we talked about it. I said: "Maybe we could give some massage to your legs and maybe that could give you a bit more strength."'

Facilitating independence. Independence was both claimed and allowed. To be independent assumed freedom from control of some sort. Patients claimed their independence and nurses allowed them to help themselves towards it. The patients were keen to develop their own level of independence, in which they could express themselves as individuals. The need for independence varied according to the unique situation of each patient. The nurses worked with the patients to find a balance between helping and not helping, so that patients were able to resume some degree of autonomous action as soon as possible.

Finding a balance in helping and not helping, so that the patient could be free to be independent, was epitomised by Jane and Max. Max appreciated the way in which Jane facilitated his independence, which was extremely precious to him. Max said:

> *'Certain people are well aware that I haven't reached my full maximum potential. I still haven't found out how far I can go...I'm just trying to maintain maximum independence...Jane quietly lets me try my own techniques first, before she intervenes. She would intervene at any time, if something went wrong.'*

Facilitating learning. Learning was important for patients and nurses. Patients were invested in their learning, because it meant that they were given the knowledge and skills to cope with the effects of their illnesses. Nurses realised that they were giving patients the tools of their freedom by making learning easier. The nurses made learning easier by the ways in which they brought their knowledge, skills and humanity to the teaching context. Teaching was a process of person to person communication, through which important information and skills were shared with patients, to enable them to cope better with their life circumstances.

The nature of the mutual investment in teaching and learning was exemplified by Peter and Jean. Jean described her diabetes education sessions with Peter, thus:

> 'I feel that Peter explains things very plain to you....He puts it in English that I can understand...It was special, because I thought that he was doing it for me...I thought he was doing it especially for me...I hope he can keep on getting through to people like he got through to me.'

Facilitating coping. The stress of illness and disability had, to varying degrees, distorted the patients' ability to manage day to day activities. For some patients, the road back to where they were originally, or to places where they had never been, represented a major journey. The path back to optimal wellbeing was made easier to traverse, as patients learned how to cope with their life circumstances. Nurses made coping easier for patients by the way they encouraged them to become proactive in finding their own level of independence and in making choices amongst alternatives.

Facilitating coping was exemplified by the interaction between Sally and Frances. Frances explained how Sally helped her after her stroke.

> 'Yes, you feel as though you are a person...You're not just rushed, you know, with a pill...I think she's very human...Tells you: "Everybody's going through it, you know and don't throw the sponge in!" You know they [the nurses] are doing it to help you, because they know, they can't be home with you all the time and if you want to go home, well, you've got to do these things.'

Facilitating comfort. For patients, a sense of comfort was integral to their everyday experience of being human. Being relatively free from various forms of psychological and physiological discomfort was welcomed, as a relief from some of the changes to their usual life patterns that their hospitalisation had caused. Nurses made the attainment of comfort easier for patients by being there, assisting them with their daily activities, and providing judicious emotional support, which was sensitive to the unique circumstances of each patient. Attending carefully to physical comfort measures often had the effect of attending simultaneously to the patient's emotional comfort.

The artistic nature of sensitivity in facilitating comfort, according to the specific needs of a patient, was demonstrated by the interaction between Sue and Becky. Becky explained how her comfort was facilitated by Sue:

> 'What I liked about the bath was it was hot. It took the pain away. It made me feel sleepy. I feel Sue's begun to give me a bit of confidence back. I had no confidence, but I...[begins to cry]...When I cry, she doesn't try to shut me up...'

Facilitating acceptance of body image changes. Sometimes recovery from an illness episode meant changes in a person's usual body structures and functioning. Whereas alterations in the body's physiological functions may have been relatively unnoticed, visible anatomical alterations presented unique challenges to patients. Waking from surgery to get accustomed to living without a leg was an event managed by each person in his or her own way. The nurses were there for patients to make the acceptance of altered body image easier. There was no prescriptive approach to facilitating acceptance of body image changes in individuals, rather, it was something which unfolded according to the unique contextual features of particular people.

The attunement to individual acceptance of altered body image was exemplified by the interaction between Sue and Naomi, in which Naomi came to gradually accept her amputated stump as part of herself. Sue described how it happened:

> 'So, I can remember the first day Naomi did it [massaged her stump]. She was so tentative. She was frightened of touching it. So, I just took her through a few basic massage techniques, and said: "It's really nice if you just give it a rub, like this..." You could see her through the day; the circles were getting bigger and bigger and bigger and more firm and the hands and the stump were an item. It wasn't a stump, that she was barely touching. It was beautiful, the way you could see it happening.'

Facilitating changes. As part of their treatment, patients were often confronted with the necessity of making considerable changes in their lifestyles. Making changes in life patterns was difficult, especially when patterns had been developed over long periods of time. Nurses made changes easier for patients by encouraging them to persist with treatment and to find ways of incorporating new ideas into their daily life. Changes began with individuals, because their cooperation was integral to them making changes successfully.

Beginning with the patient's lifestyle and facilitating changes within it, was exemplified by the interaction between Elizabeth and John. Elizabeth explained how she approached John in relation to improving his diabetic dietary habits at home.

'It was the first time I'd met him, but I read his history and he was a man who knew what he should be doing and he hadn't been doing it. I didn't want to put him on the spot, because many people have been on to him and it hasn't worked that way. I just tried to make it as informal as possible. He made a bit of a joke about his diet. He was quite amused by the fact that he likes his food and that's his trouble. I was trying to establish a friendly relationship.'

Calming fears. Illness and hospitalisation created a magnitude of fears for people, who coped with them in various ways. Fears may have been real or imagined, relatively small, or overwhelming, but they were experienced by the person and they stayed until they could be alleviated in some way. Nurses alleviated fears through explanations, general talk and company, in whatever amounts and combinations that suited particular patients' experiences.

An example of calming fears occurred in the interaction between Sally and Beryl. Beryl had been concerned about her palpitations and Sally helped to calm her fears by taking time to explain things to her. Beryl related the incident, thus:

'Well, she explained the pumping of my heart. It seems to come from my back, when I was laying down and she said if I felt like that, it would be best to sit up or put an extra pillow, because I like to lie very flat...She explained me what could ease me if I wanted, if it came on again, which is very good of her. I thought she was very nice and I liked her very much.'

Building trust. Patients submitted themselves to hospitalisation and the uncertainty that it often entailed, therefore, their new experiences presented a challenge for them, especially of putting their trust in relative strangers. Part of the patients' recovery was a reaffirmation of trust in themselves and in the world and the people around them. Nurses helped to build trust by being there with patients daily, assisting them through the stages of their illness experiences, and sharing with them as people. Nurses and patients often built trust through mutual self-disclosure, so that by showing each other something of themselves, nurses and patients began to trust each other. Peter explained:

You [the nurse] expect them [the patients] to tell you about themselves. Why shouldn't we reciprocate?...Also, always concentrating on their problems and things like that, that gets a bit wearing for both the staff and the patient, I think. Like, sometimes a general conversation, about nothing in particular, about things that happen in the paper, things that happen in the world, your history or anything like that, just like normally, if you met someone in the pub or a coffee shop or something like that [that helps].'

Giving confidence. Nurses gave patients confidence to resume their usual lives. There was no single approach that functioned routinely to give confidence, rather giving confidence was something that was orchestrated spontaneously in the daily round of activities, whenever nurses and patients interacted with one another.

Dee, who was recovering from bilateral fractured wrists, expressed the tendency of nurses to give patients confidence in this way:

> 'Whenever we [patients] call, they [nurses] are always there to help, but they get you to do things on your own too. I think I have seen so many people coming in and going, and they've improved within a couple of days...I think they just give you...more confidence in yourself and it helps you mentally and physically to get back on your feet.'

Allowing the experience to unfold. Experiences of life unfolded daily for the nurses and patients. Each day was faced for what it brought forth, and people reacted to things and interpreted them within their specific contexts. Being relatively free from preconceptions of what might have happened, and how patients might have needed to be treated, did not apply to standard technical procedures, which were a part of the care of each patient. Each patient required a certain standard of care in relation to his or her total management and that was attended to, as prescribed. However, when it came to subjective experiences, as reflected by patients' words and behaviours, there was minimal prejudgment of how patients should feel and behave.

The tendency to let an experience unfold as it would for a patient, was exemplified by Andrew and Josephine. Andrew described how he felt about Josephine's non-acceptance of being in the PNU:

> 'It was the first time I'd actually met Josephine. Yesterday, she was very unhappy about coming here, because she thought she was well enough to go home, so there was quite a bit of negativity about being in the unit. But, I mean, that's OK. There's nothing wrong with that...You've got to give them space and give them a chance to accept it, or they might never accept it fully, but just give them a chance to think about it, and [you] back off a bit.'

Summary. The aspect of facilitation illuminated the phenomenon of ordinariness in nursing by revealing some of the enabling qualities and activities of nurses and patients, whereby challenges of life were made easier for people to face. For the most part, the facilitative aspect of ordinariness in nursing flowed from nurses to patients, although nurses were also open to receive facilitative qualities and activities from patients, in various situations, in which this was appropriate.

Other things may be found to be a part of the facilitative aspect of ordinariness in nursing, however, the analysis and interpretation of the text derived from the nurse-patient interactions in this research, showed some of the relevant qualities and activities as being: appreciating skilful nursing care; appreciating help; facilitating independence; facilitating learning; facilitating coping; facilitating comfort; facilitating acceptance of body image changes; facilitating changes; calming fears; building trust; giving confidence; and allowing the experience to unfold.

Fair play

Fair play refers to the sense of reasonableness, that we possess as humans, through which we are forthright in saying what we feel we have to say, knowing that the least we can do, even partially, is to tolerate frustrating elements in others, that we recognise in ourselves. Some qualities and activities of fair play include: straight talking; and tolerating one another's humanness.

Straight talking. Speaking messages frankly and clearly occurred between nurses and patients, in situations in which one person had something to say for the benefit of the other, even though the listener may have had some difficulty in hearing it. The straight talking was returned in kind to the speaker, because the controversial nature of the talk created a reaction which also needed to be expressed. Nurses and patients expected to take turns at being both speaker and listener of straight talk. Although it risked hurt feelings, it cleared the air between the people and allowed further dialogue to ensue.

A notable example of straight talking occurred between Jane and Max. Jane gave her account of the incident, thus:

'Later on in the afternoon I went to see him [Max] and asked him about his turn [pressure care]. He said: "Oh you do what you like" and I said: "Max I don't do what I like, I do what you want me to do." "Oh," he said, "the others do this that and the other" and I said: "Where's the fight gone Max?" and he started to cry and the first thing I did was put my arms around him, because I'm a tactile person. I know if people don't want to be touched, he didn't back off he didn't freeze or anything. He just lay there.

He just stared and said: "Well you know what drugs I'm on and everything else. I've been on psychiatric drugs for so long, the psychiatrist has written me off and everything else." I said: "What a load of crap!" I said: "You go out and ask a hundred people out there and I bet they're on something to keep them going for the day." I said: "If that's the way you feel, what's the point? You're feeling sorry for yourself, that you're having to take them [drugs] to keep you going through the day." I think I floored him.

His reaction was he just 'sat' there. He said: "You're humouring me." I said: "I've never humoured you." I said: "We've always called a spade a spade." He wouldn't actually say "Yes, or no." Then afterwards he turned around and said: "Well, I've got a bit more living to do" and I said: "Good, I'm glad" so I gave him another hug.'

Tolerating one another's humanness. The more time nurses and patients took to get to know one another in the course of day to day events in the unit, the more they began to recognise human features in each other. They realised that the so-called 'roles' of patient and nurse were not scripted strictly and that each person could take the opportunity to ad lib, should the mood and the moment dictate. For instance, patients were not always long-suffering, and nurses were not always cheerful. Each person was seen as being only human, after all.

Tolerating one another's humanness was described best by Andrew, who it explained it thus:

'We're [nurses are] only human, that's right. It's probably one of the hardest jobs I know, because you've got to put it [your feelings] aside, you're supposed to. One of the things I've always found in nursing is honesty with the patient. You have some days when you come to work and you really don't want to be there and [that was] one of the things Donald [a patient] and me understood with each other. I could be really tired and I could just say to Donald: "I'm not in the mood today Donald" and those days he didn't make as many demands. I mean it's good if you can be honest with your patient. I mean Donald could be, I shouldn't say, [but he was] very demanding, but he had a lot of idiosyncrasies. Like, he always got bread, but it was toast that he wanted, not that you minded, but you know, some days you'd say you don't feel like it and you'd notice that Donald would sort of give you sort of a breather. But that was through being able to be honest with Donald. This is one of the places, working here, where I've found you can be honest with your patients, because, I suppose, of primary nursing, we've got them [the same patients] every day. A lot of the patients are here for a couple of months. You know their routine.'

Summary. Fair play included qualities and activities of straight talking and tolerating one another's humanness. It illuminated the phenomenon of ordinariness in nursing by revealing ways in which people negotiated impasses in communication, through being honest, if not somewhat blunt, yet at the same time tolerating some of the annoying features in the other person, appreciating that they too, were only human.

Familiarity

Familiarity refers to that sense we have of someone else, through the sense we have of ourselves, as individuals with a lifetime of experiences. Some qualities and activities of familiarity include: relating to one another's humanness; relating to the other's situation; acknowledging specialness in everyday situations; tolerating noisiness; relating to the patient as person; relating to the nurse as person; relating to genuineness in people; equating with a sense of 'that's all'; recognising the days in which everything seems to go wrong; and being part of everyday life.

Relating to one another's humanness. The nurses and patients shared a sense of what it was for them to be human themselves and how humanness might seem for someone else. Relating to one another's humanness was a strong bond between nurses and patients, who revealed something of themselves to one another and sensed an affinity as people living out their day to day lives in the context of the nursing unit.

An interaction between Sally and Lillian, an elderly woman recovering from a fractured hip, exemplifies the nature of relating to one another's humanness. Sally related to Lillian as a soft grandmother and Lillian related to Sally as a younger person full of help and kindness. The relationship was described in my journal, thus:

'Lillian returned from the toilet and Sally noticed how tall she looked in relation to Lillian. Sally related to Lillian as like her own 'wee granny.' Sally's remark was said with softness and received by Lillian as it was intended. It had to do with the tilt of Sally's head, her tone of voice and her smile. Lillian understood the softness in Sally's voice, just as Sally sensed Lillian's grand-motherliness.'

Relating to the other's situation. The nurses and patients understood each other in relation to the unique circumstances in which they found themselves. Although, in many cases, patients' situations were the things to which nurses related, it was not a one way pattern, rather, patients were aware of, and sensitive to, the nurses' situations.

The mutuality of relating to the other's situation was exemplified by Sally and Gus. Sally explained how Gus related to her headache.

'He sort of told me to go off and have some Panadol and make sure that I was alright and that I should look after myself and he continued to apologise...well, I think the message got across [that he didn't cause my headache], but I think that he realised that if he had a headache and someone was shouting at him [it wouldn't be too nice]...It was probably because he could put himself in my shoes.'

Acknowledging specialness in everyday situations. Nurses and patients realised that there was specialness in everyday activities, in which they engaged routinely together. Nurses acknowledged the value of time spent with patients. Accomplishing daily tasks, such as attending to hygiene needs, provided space and time for continuing dialogue and ever increasing familiarity.

Specialness in everyday situations was exemplified by an interaction between Andrew and Ruth. Ruth, who was recovering from a fractured femur, explained how Andrew transformed an everyday routine of assisting her with her shower, into something which she regarded as being special for her.

'Yes, [shower time is special, because] he's so gentle. He doesn't worry [fuss] about you. You're the patient. He looks after you. And he's Andrew and I'm the patient. And he does look after me and he looks after us all.'

Tolerating noisiness. The unit was often noisy with the traffic and clatter of everyday life, however, patients and nurses seemed to be oblivious to the noise, because they were intent on what they were doing, or because the noise was actually comfortable in a homely sort of way.

Tolerating noisiness was represented well by the interaction between Elizabeth and Joe. Elizabeth did not notice the noise and inferred through her comment that she had brought up children and was somewhat immune to noise. Joe, who seemed to take comfort in the noisiness, explained it thus:

'Yes [it is noisy], but [I feel] quite comfortable. Oh, they treat you like you're at home, I think myself...Fixing your meals up, and showering, and they help you every way they possibly can. They are all very nice people, the nurses and everything like that. That makes it bearable, yes.'

Relating to the patient as a person. The nurses related to the patients as people, who were living their own particular lives and their present circumstances, within the context of the unit. In the perception of the nurses, patients had a past, present and future, as individuals, who for the time were spending some time and space with them.

Relating to the patient as a person was exemplified by Jane, who explained how she perceived Dee:

'She is a dynamic lady and I would imagine her not stopping once she got out of here, because she's got so much energy...Probably, her bones are in far better shape than mine, because I don't exercise. She's probably far better (healthier) than I am.'

Relating to the nurse as a person. Patients related to nurses as people. Some patients were able to express what it was that they felt about the nurse as a person, whereas others simply said: 'There's something about him/her.' Naomi related to a nurse as a person, when she said this about Sue:

'Well, she seems to be such a normal sort of, she's a nurse, but as well as being a nurse, she's a friendly sort of person, who gives you confidence, I think. That makes a big difference doesn't it. You don't look at her as a clinical sort of figure altogether, she's a friend as well. It's hard to explain. Well, when I say normal, to me normal is to be friendly and helpful, as well as being that trained person, who knows what it's all about anyway, but you feel that you can talk to her as a friend. Not to be afraid to ask questions, whether it be foolish or not, because she treats you very sensibly and in a friendly manner. I just can't explain it...I don't have to be afraid of her training and because she knows so much about this and that, that I'm scared of asking her something. I don't feel like that at all. I feel I can ask her anything, sensible or not.'

Relating to genuineness in people. Genuineness was expressed separately as a quality of familiarity. A patient used the word specifically to refer to people who in his mind 'gave a damn about him.' He understood genuineness from within himself and his own experience. Patrick related to genuineness in people in this way:

'I find her [Sue] very easy to talk to. If I had a problem, or whatever, or a query, she would be the one I would see...I believe she's genuine...Well I've always considered myself a good judge of character. It's a feeling I get, that there is genuine concern. Some of the other nurses, you can tell that when you speak to them that they're not really, they're hearing you, but they're not really listening to you. When you've finished, basically it's going in one ear and out the other. They don't really give a damn.'

Equating with a sense of 'that's all'. Nurses and patients lived out a day to day existence in the unit and some of them appeared to cease to see the strangeness of the context, in comparison to their usual surroundings and lifestyles. For some patients, nursing activities, such as being washed by a nurse, or having a nurse perform an intimate procedure like a bowel evacuation, was equated with a sense of 'that's all'; or 'they are just doing their job.'

For some nurses, relatively sophisticated technical and com-municative skills were combined into interactions, which were sheer artistry to observe and, as expert practitioners, these nurses appeared to be unconscious of themselves.

Equating with a sense of 'that's all' was exemplified by Peter and Vernon. Peter tried to transcend the confines of his sense of 'that's all' by expressing the artistry of his expertise in this way:

> 'It's difficult [to explain] really. It's his [Vernon's] whole body language; the way he's trying to wash himself or not trying to wash himself. It's difficult to know, but when you look at him you just feel that he's not trying this and he doesn't particularly want to do that. I don't know what it is. It's difficult. I suppose that's what body language is all about, you just pick it up.
> She [Vernon's daughter)]may be a bit too close. She'd feel like she needs to do more for him, instead of letting him do as much as he can, when he feels that he can manage for himself and so increases his independence. I think that is the thing, where we [nurses] have to actually know when to step in and when to stand back. I think that comes with training and experience. I don't think you can just pick up someone off the street and ask them to shower somebody and expect them to do it properly.'

Vernon equated tentatively with a sense of 'that's all,' when he expressed his contradictory reactions to being washed by nurses in this way.

> *'Oh, not really [there's nothing different about Peter washing me]. You could rub me down anyway, the same as him I suppose. I sit in the chair and he does my knees and then he does my back and arms and my chest, but I wash the old personal and that's about all there is to it dear. That's all. I can do that [wash my penis]. I don't want them mucking around with that. That's what I can't understand; how all these nurses [can bear to be] mucking around with bloody old men, old droopy grubs hangin' here, there, and everywhere...*
> *Don't affect me love... Well I've had nearly every nurse in [town] wait on me. Back at my daughter's place, the District Nurses used to come out twice a week and shower me, but there was never anything spoken. I don't know you've just got to put up with it I suppose... They [the District Nurses] just treat it as a job and nothing else. A bit of love and care, they don't knock me around or anything. Everyday occurrence love.'*

Recognising the days in which everything seems to go wrong. It is said: 'Into every life, a little rain must fall' and this truism held for certain days in the unit. Recognising the days in which everything seemed to go wrong was representative of the days people wished they'd stayed in bed, because nothing, but nothing, seemed to being going well! Both Jane and Vicky had a day in which everything seemed to go wrong and it was probably summarised best in my notes:

> 'It was a day which seemed fairly joyless for the both of them. Vicky was caught up in the despair [of her hand immobility] and Jane became embroiled in a conflict of her own. Woven into Jane and Vicky's interaction that day, there was some confusion over the reporting function of the nurses in the unit. Jane expressed a gamut of emotions, when she related how Vicky's doctor threatened to transfer Vicky out of the unit. All in all, Jane and Vicky had both had a terrible day...Jane recognised that some days are not so easy to live through as others...The next day, Vicky was walking on her frame and her wailing had ceased. Jane also felt reconstituted and coped with whatever her day brought forth.'

Being part of everyday life. Nurses and patients were immersed in the daily context of the unit. It was a busy place in which people moved to and fro, continuing their interpersonal communications and creating their own community within the hospital structure.

Being part of the everyday life of the unit was exemplified in the interaction between Jane and Vicky. I recorded my observations, thus:

> 'The unit was humming with busyness that day. The motion of ward life was evident around Vicky and Jane; they wove their way in and around it as they continued their interaction...All the people interacted in their respective bubbles of reality, bumping against and merging into one another's realities as the flow of their Being-in-the-world of the unit unfolded that day. It was as though the sum total of people's experiences saturated the ambience of the unit. Regardless of their personal plights, the clamour of the day in the unit continued around them.'

Summary. The aspect of familiarity illuminated the phenomenon of ordinariness in nursing by revealing some of the qualities and activities associated with that sense we have of someone else, through the sense we have of ourselves, as individuals with a lifetime of experiences.

Other things may be a part of the familiarity aspect of ordinariness in nursing, however, the analysis and interpretation of the text derived from the nurse-patient interactions in this research, showed some of the qualities and activities as being: relating to one another's humanness; relating to the other's situation; acknowledging specialness in everyday situations; tolerating noisiness; relating to the patient as person; relating to the nurse as person; relating to each other as people; relating to genuineness in people; equating with a sense of 'that's all'; recognising the days in which everything seems to go wrong; and being part of everyday life.

Family

Family refers to the sense of home we have within ourselves, which binds us to people with whom we have blood ties or special affinities. Some qualities and activities of family include: acknowledging the relevance of family affiliations to the person; valuing the importance of home; expressing 'family-like' ties; appreciating a 'home-like' atmosphere; and preparing to go home.

Acknowledging the relevance of family affiliations to the person. The unit was a separate world from the time and space of home realities for each nurse and patient; however, family affiliations were recognised and valued within everyday dialogue between nurses and patients. In keeping family affiliations paramount, nurses and patients reminded each other of their identities as people and met each other in the middle, to bridge the gap between the artificiality of the hospital environment and the naturalness of home. Acknowledging the relevance of family and home varied for different people and their respective affiliations. For some people, family affiliations were relevant for their closeness and support; for others, the reverse seemed apparent.

The relative complexity of the relevance of family affiliations was exemplified by Alice, a woman recovering from back surgery, who explained her situation , thus:

> 'He's [my husband is] nice. He's a nice person…Out of the blue it just happened [his stroke]. You lose your husband in a sense…I know all the little things that bug me because, I can't cope with it sometimes…Roy's like a little boy. Exactly the same, like a naughty boy…Occasionally I've blow my top with him, but it doesn't help him.
>
> I suppose I've always been so independent…I had my daughter [who is now terminally ill] to fall back on and all of a sudden, you've got no-one…I've got a sister. She's had cancer. She lives in Melbourne. She can't get out of the house. She goes shopping once a week with her daughter-in-law.
>
> A brother, who has never been ill, doesn't understand at all. I didn't even tell him I was in hospital. He and his wife came. "Gee, you look well! Gosh, you do look well! Would you like a cup of tea? Are you on with the doctors or something Alice? You must be; you're in hospital all the time!" I said: "Oh yes." I've been in that many darn hospitals.'

Valuing the importance of home. Home was ever present in the day to day dialogue between nurses and patients. Patients expressed frequently the value of home for them in story telling and reminiscences, and nurses shared their thoughts of home with them also. Nurses encouraged patients to align themselves with home, and together they negotiated usual home routines associated with activities of daily living into the nursing care as often as possible.

Valuing the importance of home was exemplified in the relationship between Sally and Gus. Gus connected himself to the value of his past and present home by saying:

> 'I can't bring myself to be a city lad. I've always been a country boy. And that's all there is to it. You might have seen the [movie] picture All the Rivers Run. I have the book at home and it's a true book and all the river boats mentioned in that book are true. I don't know them all, because at the time there was about one hundred boats hanging around Echuca But only a few came up[stream] to us; the Lachlan, the Murrumbidgee and the Darling and the Edwards. Well, that's all about I can say. Then there were the passenger boats the Ruby and the Jenny...I've got a wonderful wife and a wonderful lot of girls ['chokes' with emotion] between here and my wife. I've got a lot of sweethearts. (laugh) But my wife's on top. Don't forget that! [Laugh]'

Expressing family-like ties. Sometimes the sense of family was reflected in special affinities between nurses and patients, who became so close to one another that the relationship was best expressed as a 'family-like' tie.

Expressing family-like ties was exemplified splendidly in the interaction between Andrew and Donald. Donald gave Andrew the one of the highest accolades, when he said of him:

> 'Yeah, yeah. Andrew and I get on really well together. I'd say he was more or less like a brother.'

Appreciating a home-like atmosphere. The nursing unit was structured in a homely way, to allow for relaxed interactions; however the sense of home was created by the nurses and patients within the context, so that it was a home-like context into which other health professionals and non-family members came as visitors.

Nurses and patients recognised and valued a home-like atmosphere in the Professorial Nursing Unit and this was exemplified by the interaction between Elizabeth and Joe. Joe explained his sense of the homeliness thus:

> 'Oh, they treat you like you're at home, I think myself...Fixing your meals up, and showering, and they help you every way they possibly can.'

The benefit of a home-like atmosphere was explained by Elizabeth, who was willing to have her neck massaged by a student nurse, beside Joe's bed. Elizabeth said:

'Yes, well, I needed one [a massage]. [Laugh]. But, I thought afterwards that Joe liked the friendly atmosphere, just like you do at a friend's house. I think here [in the PNU] they [the patients] treat us more as friends and equals, than they do on other wards. Yes. I think he felt comfortable in the situation.'

Preparing to go home. Even though the nursing unit was as 'home-like' as it could be, given the circumstances of people being uprooted from their usual life contexts by illness or other misfortune, the nursing unit could not, and did not, attempt to replace home as the most treasured place for people to be. Nursing care was geared towards helping people to return to their homes, if it was humanly possible. Patients prepared to go home with varying states of anticipation, depending on how they felt they would cope with their particular circumstances. Some patients realised that they would never go home again and that a nursing home would have to be a less favoured option.

Preparing to go home was exemplified by the interaction between Sue and Becky. When she went home, Becky wanted to make some changes in her life patterns, and Sue explained Becky's situation, thus:

'She [Becky] is supposed to stay in until she can fully mobilise, but because her husband wants one hundred percent attendance, I think, with this lady in particular, it will be when she is ready to go home. I can't see anyone pushing her out the door, because they [the doctors] know it [her condition] is iatrogenic [caused by medical treatment] and the nursing staff won't suggest it [going home] until she is walking around reasonably comfortably and is able to cope with her husband. She needs coping mechanisms. As she talks more people will be able to say, "Well, have you tried this or have you tried that?" She has to relearn her patterns...She has spent so much time talking about it [her problem] over the last few days that it is starting to fall into place. She knows she has to look after herself.'

Summary. The aspect of family illuminated the phenomenon of ordinariness in nursing by revealing some of the some of the qualities and activities associated with the sense of home we have within ourselves, which binds us to people with whom we have blood ties or special affinities.

Other things may be a part of the family aspect of ordinariness in nursing, however, the analysis and interpretation of the text derived from the nurse-patient interactions in this research, showed some of the qualities and activities as being: acknowledging the relevance of family affiliations to the person—husband, wife, son, daughter, grandson, granddaughter, brother, sister; valuing the importance of home; expressing family-like ties; appreciating a home-like atmosphere; and preparing to go home.

Favouring

Favouring refers to the approval we give to other people and ourselves for commendable qualities, which remind us of our essential nature as human beings. Some qualities and activities of favouring include approving commendable human qualities and enjoying statements of appreciation.

Approving commendable human qualities. Patients and nurses recognised and approved commendable human qualities in each other, such as goodness, niceness, loveliness, friendliness, helpfulness, kindness, caring, and gentleness. The qualities were often expressed without further elaboration, as though extra words could not say more than could be said by a carefully chosen definitive adjective, or set of adjectives. The expressions of approval revealed an affinity of liking and appreciation between patients and nurses, and in affirming those qualities within others, each reaffirmed those qualities within themselves.

Approving commendable human qualities was exemplified by Vernon, who said of Peter:

> 'He's [Peter is] a good man, a helluva good man. I've got no gripes, I'm quite happy with him...He's a very gentle man, Peter. He knows every move you should make and he makes you do it, that's what I like about him...It's his nature. Peter is a gentle man...Peter doesn't hurry you. He just says: "Say when you're ready. Sing out." Nice lad that one.'

Enjoying statements of appreciation. Nurses worked daily with people, doing their jobs to the best of their abilities and not expecting to receive statements of appreciation in return. When they received a compliment, however, nurses accepted it, often fairly coyly, but always with pleasure. Elizabeth explained her pleasure in receiving statements of appreciation from Mary, a woman who was recovering following a below knee amputation.

> 'I was quite pleased that she chose me [to take over her care]. She said she'd seen me interact with the patient across the room and she felt quite comfortable with me. That was nice to think that she felt that way...[It made me feel] good, naturally. Everybody likes a compliment.'

Summary. The aspect of favouring illuminated the phenomenon of ordinariness in nursing by revealing some of the some of the qualities and activities associated with the approval we give to other people and ourselves for commendable qualities, which remind us of our essential nature as human beings.

Other things may be a part of the favouring aspect of ordinariness in nursing, however the analysis and interpretation of the text derived from the nurse-patient interactions in this research showed some of the qualities and activities as being approving commendable human qualities and enjoying statements of appreciation.

Feelings

Feelings refers to the way we sense ourselves in relation to our worlds of people and things; sometimes as feeling high, sometimes as feeling low, sometimes as feeling somewhere in between. Some qualities and activities of feelings include: acknowledging the polarity of human feelings; and expressing feelings.

Acknowledging the polarity of human feelings. In their day to day lives in the nursing unit, nurses and patients acknowledged the polarity of their human feelings. Depending on what was happening for each individual, nurses and patients acknowledged the presence in themselves and others, of the full gamut of human feelings, including being happy or sad, being in comfort or pain, being relaxed or agitated, being calm or in fear and being angry or content.

An especially poignant example of the polarity of human feelings was expressed by Ellen, who enjoyed sharing a sense of fun with Jane, but who nevertheless understood her own feelings in a seemingly contradictory way.

> 'She was helping me put my bras on and a bit of powder and I said: "Wait for my flaps [breasts]." Jane laughed, oh she laughed! She had to stop work for a while. You know, we get on sort of well. She's got a good sense of humour and I have…Oh well, she's such a happy person. I enjoy her. We have a joke, when I have a wash. When I want a bit of powder on, I put it on my wee flaps. The wash is a little bit of a joke, you know. She's a lovely girl, she is, a great sense of humour.
>
> But you know, I can't laugh. It is funny, I can't laugh. I don't know. The only thing that makes me laugh is a [movie] picture, not a funny one, it's got to be a stupid one, a really stupid English one. Some pictures are just really stupid you know and I'll just laugh. I don't laugh and I don't cry…It seems that I just can't! Even when my husband was killed, I don't think I shed a tear.'

Expressing feelings. Having feelings, and actually expressing them, can be two different things. Nurses and patients gave voice to their feelings in relation to all sorts of things, about whatever was of interest to them, according to the particular situations in which they found themselves. Nurses and patients understood that there was full license to express their feelings and some availed themselves of the opportunities. Sue exemplified the value of expressing feelings, when she described her perceptions of massaging Ralph, a man who was undergoing detoxification of alcohol, thus:

'It seems weird, when we talk about giving enemas and shaving people and that, but massage is probably one of the most intimate things we do with patients, because it creates the most intimate responses. And with Ralph, he just felt really calm, relaxed. I don't think he was genuine in his reactions [during the interaction when the researcher was present], like, if it had just been the two of us here, just purely done a massage, I think different aspects would have come out, because I would have literally shut up then and just let him talk, but he was aware that he had two people there and he was interacting with both. But he didn't seem at all perturbed about sharing what he was feeling, what he was going through. I couldn't feel any tension when I asked specific questions. I couldn't feel any muscle tension coming through. He just seemed very relaxed with the both of us being there, very comfortable. When you think of it, it is so intimate to have someone laying hands on you.'

Summary. The aspect of feelings illuminated the phenomenon of ordinariness in nursing by revealing some of the some of the qualities and activities associated with sensing ourselves in relation to our worlds of people and things; sometimes as feeling high, sometimes as feeling low, sometimes as feeling somewhere in between.

Other things may be a part of the feelings aspect of ordinariness in nursing, however the analysis and interpretation of the text derived from the nurse-patient interactions in this research, showed some of the qualities and activities as being acknowledging the polarity of human feelings and expressing feelings.

Fun

Fun refers to a sense of merriment, which lightens our day to day lives and reacquaints us with the child within us all. Fun includes enjoying a sense of humour.

Enjoying a sense of humour. Nurses and patients exhibited their enjoyment of a sense of humour by laughing, joking, cheekiness, and general happiness. Enjoying a sense of humour permeated the entire nursing unit, to the extent that even people in pain and distress appreciated a well placed light word or joke. It was as though humour softened the hard realities of people's circumstances and provided a means of levity, albeit temporarily, above the inevitability of certain ultimate tragedies. Humour was always shared, never imposed. Humour was always sensitive to the other's situation and reached across the gap of the separate existence of nurses and patients, to seal their common humanity with a shared sense of merriment.

The aspect of fun is probably exemplified best by choosing one interaction for each of the nurses, which shows the qualities and activities associated with a sense of humour, although there are many more. Donald said this in relation to Andrew:

> 'He was always very jovial. We used to give one another a lot of cheek about football. Andrew was Essendon I was Collingwood and we used to throw a lot of rubbish at one another. Yeah, we'd have a great discussion about it.'

Mary said this in relation to Elizabeth:

> 'I have a knee sore [an amputated leg], so I had stitches in it and so it's about an inch apart the stitches, and so we always make fun. I had a brother that was always doing bad needle sewing. I always said it reminds me of him. We make fun of it each time she looks to see.'

I made this summary in relation to Jane and Max:

> 'The focus of their interaction was a very intimate procedure, which had its amusing side. The regular bowel evacuation procedure, which Jane and Max undertook together, was a well known event amongst the nursing staff on the unit. It had been symbolised in the form of a joke amongst the nursing staff; a chocolate box containing a piece of fake faeces, which was presented to Jane at a staff party. Jane decided to share the joke with Max and presented the box to him the next time the bowel evacuation procedure was due to be done. He knew the presentation was coming; it was a 'set up job,' but he went along with it, because it was fun and he knew that Jane knew how he would react.'

I made this summary in relation to Peter and Vernon:

> '[During the shower] Peter offers to wash Vernon's hair. As he is lathering the soap into Vernon's hair, Peter comments on

his lack of hair. A few brief words are exchanged and then Vernon looks at Peter and says: "You have a small head." By this time Peter is wiping Vernon elsewhere and quips: "Thank you very much Vernon. I love you too!" They both laugh. This is tit for tat, in a light hearted exchange.'

Gus said this in relation to Sophie and Sally:

'As I say, I have a lot of fun with them. I know I'm a bit cheeky sometimes, but I have a lot of fun with them.'

Ralph said this in relation to Sue:

'So I said to Sue, whose nails weren't all that short before she started: "Let's have a look at your nails," jokingly, because she's five stone heavier than me! So she jokingly said: "They're alright." With that over, we proceeded. So she said: "He's been reading up. He's checking on me." Oh no, [I was] quite at ease. I was looking forward to it. That's why I thought I'd better read up a bit on this massage business, just so I could sling off and try and find something wrong with the deal on the way through, but I couldn't, so...'

Summary. The aspect of fun illuminated the phenomenon of ordinariness in nursing by revealing some of the some of the qualities and activities associated a sense of merriment, which lightens our day to day lives and reacquaints us with the child within us all. Other things may be a part of the fun aspect of ordinariness in nursing, however the analysis and interpretation of the text derived from the nurse-patient interactions in this research showed that fun included enjoying a sense of humour.

Friendship

Friendship refers to knowing people well enough to regard them with affection. Some qualities and activities of friendship include: acknowledging the importance of company and talking; expressing affection and liking, and taking time to know one another.

Acknowledging the importance of company and talking. Nurses and patients spent many hours together in the nursing unit, and they acknowledged the value of being there for one another for companionship and support. Patients valued especially the time nurses spent with them talking and just spending time generally. Nurses understood that sometimes company and talking was the most they could provide, as well as assisting people with their activities of everyday living.

Acknowledging the importance of company and talking was shown in the interaction between Sally, Sophie and Gus. Gus explained it, thus:

> 'Well, myself, I found it [the conversation with Sally] good. I mean to say, she's a busy girl and I could talk to her all day and all night. Do you know what I mean? Well, they'll [the nurses will] do anything for you, to help you. Anytime. I could sit here all night and I'd still get my cups of tea or coffee and all that. They'd come in at night time, 'cause I'd be in trouble at night time. I used to prop that [the amputated leg] and make a noise some nights. They'd hear me, and they'd come in and say "I don't think that this [the phantom pain] can be fixed." It's gotta just take it's own course, I think.'

Expressing affection and liking. Some nurses and patients knew each other so well that they felt and expressed affection and liking for each other. Affection came from catching glimpses of each other as people, whose many human similarities far outweighed their differences as patients and nurses, in terms of professional knowledge and skill. Affection and liking towards one another extended past the world of the nursing unit to connections with each other after the period of hospitalisation. Close ties with patients created some personal emotional risks for nurses, especially as some patients would continue to be admitted until they finally succumbed to their disease in death.

Expressing affection and liking were expressed aptly by Andrew, who explained some special relationships with patients, thus:

> 'It [friendship] is nice, it gets hard at times too. Well, again with Donald and Kevin, another patient, they both went down hill once and that's when it becomes very hard, because you almost feel part of the family. We rang the patients up on Christmas day and it's amazing. It is like you're part of the family and you go round the houses and see them, just the way you're treated. So when something does go wrong, I shouldn't say you feel it more, or maybe you do feel it more…Donald could go in and out a couple of times, Kevin will probably come in and stay.'

Taking time to know one another. The nursing unit was a setting in which many people came to know one another well. Depending on the time span and frequency of interactions, patients and nurses knew one another to varying degrees. The time patients and nurses spent together was interrupted, even though primary nursing provided some continuity in nursing care. Being shift workers, nurses came to the unit and went home daily, took days off, and went on holidays, and patients recovered and went home, were transferred elsewhere, or died.

Time and opportunity created differences in the ways nurses and patients were able to get to know one another, however, intensive efforts were made to shorten the introductory periods of relationships, so that people could get to know one another as well as possible, in whatever time was available. For the nurses, there was much to know about patients, not only about their experiences of their illnesses, but also about who and how they were as people with social networks and individual hopes and fears.

Sally exemplified taking time to get to know one another, when she expressed her relationship with Lillian, another patient, thus:

'With Lillian, the first week I thought: "Oh, this lady's deaf" and she didn't seem interested. I sort of didn't worry about it the first night and then, the next time I met her, was last night and I started talking to her and spoke a bit louder, because she didn't have her hearing aid and she started chatting away and telling me how she went off to day hospital and likes to be active and I thought: "This lady is just getting isolated because of her hearing problem," and that was more of a reason to put a little bit more of an effort in, because I could leave her out just because of that. Once I was aware of it I thought I would make a point of actually talking to her each night, just say something to her. I mean I don't know her very well, but, the little bit I know about her is that the more opportunity I give her and the more time I spend with her, the more she's going to open up.'

Summary. The aspect of friendship illuminates the phenomenon of ordinariness in nursing by revealing some of the some of the qualities and activities associated with knowing people well enough to regard them with affection. Other things may be a part of the friendship aspect of ordinariness in nursing, however the analysis and interpretation of the text derived from the nurse-patient interactions in this research, showed some of the qualities and activities as being: acknowledging the importance of company and talking; expressing affection and liking, and taking time to know one another.

In the section above, I introduced and described the eight aspects that illuminated something of the nature of the phenomenon of ordinariness in nursing. These were: facilitation; fair play; familiarity; family; favouring; feelings; fun and friendship. As I mentioned previously, I realised at this point that the research had not gone far enough in explicating the ontological nature of the phenomenon, so I had to move beyond this point to somewhere else.

The actualities

As I have explained, the externalised qualities and activities of the phenomenon formed the aspects that have been described, and these gave some direct illumination to the phenomenon of ordinariness in nursing. To extend the gemstones metaphor that I used previously, I found that I had to crack open the aspects to see what resided within them. I coined the term 'actualities' to represent what Husserl called 'essences' and what Heidegger called 'Dasein,' or 'There-Being.' I chose the term to express the innermost identities of the aspects, because it seemed to me to be more user-friendly for the nurses and patients, who embodied ordinariness, as well as for all of those people who might seek to understand something of Being through reading the research.

The ontological nature of ordinariness in nursing was the nature within the aspects illuminating the phenomenon; that is, it was at the level of its actualities: within facilitation there was 'allowingness'; within fair play there was 'straightforwardness'; within familiarity there was 'self-likeness'; within family there was 'homeliness'; within favouring there was 'favourableness'; within feelings there was 'intuneness,' within fun there was 'lightheartedness' and within friendship there was 'connectedness.'

When I sought to describe the nature of 'allowingness', 'straightforwardness', 'self-likeness', 'homeliness', 'favourableness', 'intuneness', 'lightheartedness', and 'connectedness', I found that a clearer image of the nature of ordinariness in nursing emerged. Each one of the actualities had its own features, and each was reflective of the image of Being, as it was represented by the human qualities of the people involved in the nursing encounters. I realised that these images were context-dependent, as is the case with any meanings that emerge from interpretive research methods such as phenomenology. I acknowledged that the actualities showed themselves as how they were at that time, in that light, to that researcher, given research features such as the time, space, and organisational factors of its setting, participants and methods. I knew that I could not claim generalisability to other settings and people, nor would I want to; however, it seemed that the closer I moved to the centre of the 'gems' by explicating their actualities, the more I saw the homogeneity of the human condition unfolding as potentiating energy in front of my eyes. I trust that the following descriptions of the actualities will explain what I mean by this claim of the sameness of humanity.

Allowingness. This is an actuality of the phenomenon of ordinariness, within which people try to make things easier for other people. In nursing, allowingness creates the potential for patients and nurses to help themselves, by providing some guidance and support until such a time, if at all, that people feel able to take over their own daily life business. Allowingness is considerate of the other person's needs to be independent and dignified; it helps quietly and carefully, always attentive to the cues within the other person, that suggest a preparedness to resume increasingly autonomous thoughts and actions. Allowingness knows the other for whom it seeks facilitation, because it knows its own enabling nature as part of itself. Allowingness is an actuality of being human, therefore it recognises itself in another human and relates to other person through sensitive helping.

Straightforwardness. This is an actuality of the phenomenon of ordinariness, within which people express their thoughts, in relation to others. In nursing, straightforwardness creates the potential for patients and nurses to speak to each other as frankly as possible, saying whatever it is that is in need of being said, at the same time tolerating each other's humanness. Straightforwardness is clear and concise in its delivery and generous in its intent; it speaks to the other to unblock impasses and puts the perceived focus of contention plainly on view, to trigger discussion. Straightforwardness knows the other for whom it seeks fair play, because it knows its own frank nature as part of itself. Straightforwardness is an actuality of being human, therefore it recognises itself in another human and relates to that person through sensitive straight talking.

Self-likeness. This is an actuality of the phenomenon of ordinariness, within which people see themselves mirrored, to some degree, in other people. In nursing, self-likeness creates the potential for patients and nurses to understand the humanness of themselves in others, sharing an affinity as humans together, who are bonded by the commonality of their ordinary human existence. Self-likeness is the glue of oneness, wherein people share a sense of togetherness, regardless of a vicissitude of differences; it is a source of recognition of Being within human beings, a sense of the ultimate sameness of all people and things in the Universe. Self-likeness knows the other for whom it seeks familiarity, because it knows its own human nature as part of itself. Self-likeness is an actuality of being human, therefore, it recognises itself in another human and relates to that person through sensitive relating.

Homeliness. This is an actuality of the phenomenon of ordinariness, within which we regard people as family, either through blood ties or special affinities. In nursing, homeliness creates the potential for patients and nurses to develop close interpersonal relationships, that encompass perspectives of people as family. Homeliness is sharing common understandings with people, and in so doing, accepting a share of their joys and pains, which are integral to closer human relationships. Homeliness knows the other for whom it is family, because it knows its own bonding nature as part of itself. Homeliness is an actuality of being human, therefore it recognises itself in another human and relates to that person through sensitive family bonding.

Favourableness. This is an actuality of the phenomenon of ordinariness, within which we are reminded of our own commendable qualities by seeing them in other people, as a mirror of our essential nature as human beings. In nursing, favourableness creates the potential for patients and nurses to give approval to other people and themselves, and in so doing, to magnify the attractive aspects of themselves. Favourableness is seeing beauty in people at the inside level; it recognises everyday human qualities that defy adequate description, and realises that it is only through sensing them within itself, that it is able to know that these qualities exist and how they are. Favourableness knows the other for whom it seeks to give favour, because it knows its own pleasing nature as part of itself. Favourableness is an actuality of being human, therefore it recognises itself in another human and relates to that person through sensitive favouring.

Intuneness. This is an actuality of the phenomenon of ordinariness, within which we are sensitive to our feelings, and find licence to express them as a legitimate part of ourselves and the polarity of things within our worlds. In nursing, intuneness creates the potential for patients and nurses to acknowledge and express the polarity of their feelings. Intuneness is clearing away the debris of rationality to face up to, and embrace, the rawness of emotions, which when expressed, unblock the streams of human reactivity and cause our life energies to flow a little easier. Intuneness knows the other with whom it seeks to share its feelings, because it knows its own feeling nature as part of itself. Intuneness is an actuality of being human, therefore, it recognises itself in another human and relates to that person through sensitive expressions of feeling.

Lightheartedness. This is an actuality of the phenomenon of ordinariness, within which we share our sense of fun. In nursing, lightheartedness creates the potential for patients and nurses to express themselves though humour. Lightheartedness is levity above the everyday circumstances that cloud our minds and weigh our bodies down. Lightheartedness seeks to aerate the lead ball of life and turn it into a bright balloon. Lightheartedness knows the other for whom it seeks humour, because it knows its own laughing nature as part of itself. Lightheartedness is an actuality of being human, therefore it recognises itself in another human and relates to that person through sensitive humouring.

Connectedness. This is an actuality of the phenomenon of ordinariness, within which we sense ourselves as friends. In nursing, connectedness creates the potential for patients and nurses to know one another well enough to regard each other with affection. Connectedness is recognising friendly aspects in other people and coming in closer to get to know them. Connectedness takes time to get to know the other person, through keeping company and talking. Connectedness knows the other with whom it seeks friendship, because it knows its own befriending nature as part of itself. Connectedness is an actuality of being human, therefore it recognises itself in another human and relates to that person through sensitive liking.

The actualities were expressed as potentiating energies within the aspects of ordinariness, rather like the energy of the vacuum, or the generativity of the void. In the end, though, I realised that I had found more words to express what I believe is unexpressable in this dimension, that elusive thing called Being. I knew that I was far from the first person to experience the 'ungraspability' of Being as a concept. Heidegger knew the frustration of a lifelong search for explicating Being, resorting as he did finally, after many years of ontological enquiry, to naming Being, 'Es' (Itself).

The effects of ordinariness: the qualities and activities of its aspects

In considering the effects of the phenomenon, I returned to an important methodological assumption of phenomenology, which asserts that in order to know the nature of the thing of interest, one goes to the thing itself. If one goes to the phenomenon and searches out its nature, and if one can assume that one indeed has illuminated the thing intended, the effects of its nature can only be the effects of the thing itself; it cannot be anything else other than itself. This line of reasoning is in line with Heidegger (1962 trans.), who was unable to explicate Being through a temporal analysis, however he referred to Being as Es (Itself). Therefore, if Being is Itself, it can be nothing else.

Using this reasoning, I remembered that I had moved from the place and people features of the research context to find the nature of the phenomenon, so I decided that it was now necessary to move 'backwards,' from the phenomenon towards the research context, in order to locate the effects. I imagined Being as residing within context, and context as residing within Being. To me, they became one in the same and they could not be something different from one another; therefore, I supposed that the nature of the phenomenon reflected its effects. I conceptualised the move from context to phenomenon, to find the nature of the thing, and the move from phenomenon to context, to find the effects of the thing, as a mirror image. The nature of the phenomenon within the actualities of the phenomenon reflected back towards the qualities and activities as effects that emerged out of the context. This logic being reasonable, it then followed that the effects of the phenomenon of ordinariness in nursing were those very qualities and activities that comprised the aspects of the phenomenon.

Through the various ways of expressing human embodiment in nursing situations, all of these effects have the potential of enhancing nursing encounters. The effects of ordinariness in nursing increase the quality of the nurse-patient relationship, thereby potentiating its therapeutic effects. The enhancement of the nurse-patient relationship is described in the section that follows.

Enhancement through aspect and actuality

Facilitation and allowingness. The nursing encounter is enhanced through facilitation and allowingness. There is reciprocity in allowingness, although the flow of facilitation is determined by who has the need, and how much need there is, as well as who is in the best position to make the other's challenge easier to face. In nursing encounters, patients often have the greatest need for help because of their illness circumstances; however, patients can facilitate nurses' needs through their allowingness, especially in the effects of appreciating help; facilitating learning; facilitating coping; facilitating comfort; facilitating changes; calming fears; building trust; giving confidence; and allowing the experience to unfold.

Fair play and straightforwardness. Straightforwardness enhances nursing encounters by freeing nurses and patients to speak their minds clearly and plainly, having taken into account the relative strengths and weaknesses of their own human condition, before dispensing their straight talking to the other person. The enhancement of nursing encounters is through the frankness and forthrightness of the speaking, and the reactive freedom of the listening. When nurses and patients know each other well enough to share straight talking, they know each other well enough to risk a friendship worth keeping; therefore, nursing encounters are enhanced through nurses and patients being at that level of rapport that allows straightforwardness to express itself.

Familiarity and self-likeness. The nursing encounter is enhanced through self-likeness, because nurses and patients have a means of recognising themselves in one another. Self-likeness raises the possibilities of nurses and patients relating, acknowledging, equating, recognising, and being part of their respective worlds, through a shared sense of being human. Whilst recognising and respecting the different talents each person brings to nursing encounters, patients and nurses are connected more by their similarities as humans than they are disconnected by their differences as clients and professionals respectively.

Family and homeliness. Nursing encounters are enhanced through homeliness, because it affords the possibilities of acknowledging, valuing, expressing, appreciating, and preparing for treasured qualities and activities in relation to family and home. Homeliness centres nurses and patients inwardly with a sense of home and belonging, through blood ties or special affinities, because it creates strong bonds between them, allowing the potential of greater self-growth, from a personal base made stronger through feelings of inner security and family-like relationships.

Favouring and favourableness. Favourableness is the recognition and endorsement of human qualities, as an expression of human nature. Favourableness enhances nursing encounters by approving and enjoying commendable human qualities in oneself and others. When human qualities are recognised and approved by nurses and patients, they have the potentiality of bringing out a stronger alignment with these positive human qualities, thus creating further enhancement of nursing encounters.

Feelings and intuneness. Mutual acknowledgment and expression of feelings enhances the nursing encounter by reaffirming the shared sense of reactivity to the polar existence of living life as human beings. Enhancement of nursing encounters comes about through nurses and patients sensing that life is about highs and lows and in-betweens, and realising that it is reasonable to acknowledge and express these feelings to themselves and to others.

Fun and lightheartedness. There is mutual enjoyment in lightheartedness, as nurses and patients invite one another to take a brief respite from the heaviness of their circumstances, to be lifted momentarily by some light relief. Nursing encounters are enhanced through sharing the surprise of humour and revisiting the child within, by virtue of its transitory liberating and lightening effects.

Friendship and connectedness. There is mutual acknowledgment and expression in connectedness, with the potential for ever increasing bonds of friendship, through knowing one another over time. Enhancement of nursing encounters occurs through connectedness, when nurses and patients step outside their patient-nurse roles, which favour distancing and detachment, to risk the vulnerability of closeness for the therapeutic effects of friendship that it brings.

The nature of ordinariness in nursing was explored by moving conceptually from the research context towards the actualities of the phenomenon. Conversely, the effects of ordinariness in nursing were described by beginning with the actualities and moving back towards the research context. The rationale for doing this was that the phenomenon of ordinariness in nursing is what it is, it can be nothing else but itself; therefore, its nature and effects are one in the same phenomenon, as images of one another. Each of the aspects and their respective actualities has the potential to increase the quality of the nurse-patient relationship, thus potentiating the therapeutic effects of nursing encounters when nurses and patients feel free to be themselves in the relatively strange contexts of health care settings.

10. A redefinition of nursing

In the concluding chapter of this book I will describe some possibilities of ordinariness for nurses and other health care professionals, before I offer a redefinition of nursing based on the insights of the research into ordinariness in nursing. The redefinition is simplicity itself, because it relates to the people-oriented, everyday work of nursing. The concluding section will extend the original findings of the research to suggest an extension which is actually an ancient awareness, and this is that humans are spirit-filled beings, who are united in the extraordinary potential of their ordinariness.

Some possibilities of ordinariness for nursing practice

Ordinariness presents some possibilities for nurses and other health care professionals, who find personally that there is relevance for them in these research findings. The research found that nurses and patients shared a common sense of humanity. Within the context of caring, the nurses were ordinary people, perceived as being extraordinarily effective by the very ways in which their humanness shone through their knowledge and skills, to make their whole being with patients something more than just professional helping.

The patients attuned themselves with the nurses, because of their sense of affinity with the nurses as humans. At the same time, the patients acknowledged the nurses' knowledge and skills and allowed themselves to be supported by the nurses' professional qualities and activities. The shared sense of ordinariness between nurses and patients made them as one in their humanness and created a special place, in which the relative strangeness of the experience of being in a health care setting could be made familiar and manageable.

Nurses are involved in day to day practice, interacting most frequently and intimately with patients; therefore, nurses who recognise the appropriateness of the meanings may find some possibilities for enhancing the therapeutic value of their practice. Each of the aspects of the phenomenon contained qualities and activities that could have applications for other nurses in their daily practice. These possibilities will be raised in the section that follows.

Some practice possibilities of facilitation

When nurses are able to work skilfully, informed by the ever growing knowledge base of their professional education and their clinical experiences, tasks and people become combined into a pattern of seemingly effortless actions, which flow according to the needs of each particular situation. Nurses can help and be helped in nursing. Being consciously alert to, and in tune with, the unique contextual features of nurse-patient interactions can create the potential for facilitative acts of caring between nurses and patients.

Patients require varying degrees of help from nurses, and some of them are willing to express their need for help; others are hesitant to request help, while others rely entirely on the nurses to be in tune with any help they need. When nurses negotiate with patients in planning their daily activities, the matching of each person's needs to the help they require can be achieved by sensitivity to that individual. The sensitivity to monitoring a person's need for help can be fine tuned by taking time in getting to know them well enough to be able to offer help appropriate to their needs. This fine tuning constitutes an artistic practice in nursing, which comes with practice experience.

Patient independence is both claimed and allowed, therefore it assumes freedom from control of some sort. When patients claim their independence and nurses allow them to help themselves towards it, some degree of autonomous patient action is possible, even in situations that appear to be constraining. Nurses can be aware that, in order for patients to assert their independence, nurses may need to encourage its expression in patients, and nurses can become aware of, and attempt to remove, various controlling influences that may be constraining patients' expressions of independence.

The path back to optimal wellbeing is made easier to follow as patients learn how to cope with their life circumstances. Nurses make coping easier for patients by encouraging them to become proactive in finding their own level of independence and in making choices amongst alternatives. Nurses can realise that the source of coping resides in patients, and that they act as facilitators of those coping behaviours and attitudes, by assisting patients in locating, and choosing among, their own life choices.

Nurses give patients the tools of their freedom, by making learning easier. Nurses can make learning easier by the ways in which they bring their knowledge, skills and humanity to the teaching context, in a process of person to person communication through which important information and skills can be shared with patients, to enable them to cope better with their life circumstances. This type of instruction is geared to the person in a way that makes comprehensible those things that need to be learned. Teaching then becomes more than matching of the content to the person; it also involves careful attention to the quality of the human relationship through which the knowledge and skills are shared.

Nurses can make the attainment of comfort easier for patients by being there, assisting them with their daily activities, and by providing judicious emotional support, which is sensitive to the unique circumstances of each patient. Nurses can realise that attending carefully to physical comfort measures can often have the effect of simultaneously attending to the patient's emotional comfort.

When nurses are there for patients, it makes the acceptance of altered body image somehow easier. There is no prescriptive approach to facilitating the acceptance of body image changes in individuals; rather, it is an attunement of nurse and patient, which unfolds according to the unique contextual features of particular people. There is a special knowing that comes from daily interaction, that creates opportunities for small gestures, such as a word here and there, a look, a suggestion of help to cope, and so on. These things cannot be prescribed into an ordered account of failsafe methods for assisting in the acceptance of body image changes, rather they are things which happen between people, who are sensitive to the subtle changes in daily progress and who are there, ready to offer whatever is necessary, in that moment of caring.

Nurses can make changes easier for patients by encouraging them to persist with treatment and to find ways of incorporating new ideas into their daily life. Nurses need to realise that changes in patients begin with those individuals and their co-operation is integral to them making their particular changes successfully. In this way, changes are negotiated—not imposed.

Illness and hospitalisation create a magnitude of fears for people and nurses can help to alleviate patients' fears through explanations, and general talk and company, in whatever amounts and combinations that suit the particular patients' experiences. Nurses can realise that small things matter, like tea and talk, because they provide enormous benefits such as time and company, which indicate to patients nurses' willingness to take time to be with them.

Nurses help to build trust by being there with patients daily, assisting them through the stages of their illness experiences and sharing with them as people. Nurses and patients can build trust through mutual self-disclosure, by showing each other something of their own personal selves, even though, ostensibly, the setting is professional. Nurses require so much personal information from patients, and in a professional relationship it might be accepted that this sharing is always unilateral. In their willingness to share something of themselves through sensitive and appropriate self disclosure, however, nurses can demonstrate the reciprocal nature of trust.

Nurses can give patients confidence to resume their usual lives. There is no singular approach which functions to give confidence, rather giving confidence is something that is orchestrated spontaneously in the daily round of activities, whenever nurses and patients interact sensitively with one another.

When each day is faced for what it brings forth, and people react to things from moment to moment, within their specific contexts, nurses can be relatively free from preconceptions and have minimal prejudgment of how patients 'should' feel and behave. This freedom from prejudgment does not apply to standard technical procedures, which are a part of the care of each patient and require a certain standard of care that must be attended to, as prescribed. However, in instances when prejudicial reactions are possible, nurses can consider the uniqueness of people and their situations, and have no particular judgements, other than people have the right to make their own choices.

Some practice possibilities of fair play

When messages are spoken frankly and clearly between nurses and patients, in situations in which one person has something to say for the benefit of the other, even though the listener may have some difficulty in hearing it, the controversial nature of the talk can create a reaction, which also needs to be expressed. If nurses and patients take turns at being both speaker and listener of straight talk, it has the potential to clear the air between them and allow further dialogue to ensue. Nurses and patients are only prepared to speak to each other in this way if they know one another well enough to speak plainly and frankly. A relationship such as this takes time to foster.

When nurses and patients get to know one another in the course of their day to day events, they can begin to recognise human features in each other. When they realise that the so-called 'roles' of long-suffering patient and all-helpful nurse are not strictly scripted, and that each person can take the opportunity to ad lib, as the mood and the moment dictates, they can learn to tolerate one another's 'only human' side in a way that allows further personal progress.

Some practice possibilities of familiarity

If nurses and patients share a sense of what it is for them to be human themselves, and how humanness might seem for someone else, they can relate to one another's humanness and share a sense of affinity, as people living out their day to day lives in the context of a nursing setting. Nurses need to realise that the sense of humanness begins with themselves; therefore, they need to allow themselves to acknowledge and surface their humanness, and to let it come through in their professional interactions.

When nurses and patients understand each other in relation to their unique circumstances, they can relate to each other's situations. Nurses can create specialness in everyday activities, by providing space and time for continuing dialogue and ever increasing familiarity with patients. Time and opportunity for interpersonal communication are essential for the development of effective nurse-patient relationships. Nurses can choose to make the development of interpersonal relationships a high priority in their daily work activities and processes.

It may be important to consider sometimes that patients and nurses might be oblivious to the noise of the traffic and clatter of everyday life in nursing settings, because they are either intent on what they are doing, or the noise is actually comfortable in a homely sort of way. The possibilities in this awareness are related to creating, or allowing, a friendly, albeit somewhat noisy atmosphere for patients sometimes, when this seems appropriate.

When nurses relate to patients as people, they can begin to see them as individuals, who are living their own particular lives and circumstances. Thus, nurses can relate to patients as people, who have a past, present and future, and respect them as people, who are sharing some time and space with them. In this way, patients become seen as people in their own rights, and not just diagnostic labels and responsibilities.

Patients can relate to nurses as people and sometimes patients are able to express what it is that they feel about a nurse as person, whereas sometimes they simply say: 'There's something about her', or 'him'. The possibilities for practice here are related to the awareness that patients may not always express how they feel, but that they are impressed when they make the personal discovery that the nurse is a person, just like themselves. When this happens, nurses become seen as people in their own right, and not just the dispensers of professional help.

Patients are able to sense genuineness in nurses. They can differentiate quite readily between those nurses who are just doing their job, and those nurses who 'give a damn about them.' The message for nurses in this realisation is that nurses need to value patients as perceptive beings, who are willing and able to share their perceptions.

Some nurses may be relatively unaware of the sophisticated technical and communicative skills they have as expert practitioners. Nurses need to take time to think about their nursing practice. Reflection on nursing practice allows nurses to transcend the confines of their own taken-for-granted sense of 'that's all' there is to nursing, to describe the sophisticated science and artistry of their practice.

Everyone can experience bad days. Life brings its low points and days where everything seems to go wrong. Nurses can recognise that they can work through bad days, knowing that they will have an end. This relates to the expectations that some people might hold that, for days to go well, they need to appear to be mostly of a positive nature. Lessons may be learned in uncomfortable situations, and the acknowledgment that bad days are reasonably expected and negotiated, can be instructive for patients and nurses alike.

Nurses and patients create their own community within the hospital structure, by their immersion in the daily activities of nursing. The life of health care settings goes on in and around nurse-patient interactions and the ambience of the wards can become saturated with noise, movement and interpersonal communications. The possibilities for practice here are related to nurses tuning their awareness into the clinical clamour, so that it can be experienced clearly in all its intricacies, reflected on, and sometimes adjusted spontaneously, while the nurse is an active part of it all. The reflection-in-action then becomes a source of awareness and possible change of attitudes and behaviours.

Some possibilities of family

When nurses keep family affiliations paramount, nurses and patients can remind each other of their identities as people, and meet each other in the middle, to bridge the gap between the artificiality of the hospital environment and the naturalness of home. Nursing settings can be structured in homely ways, to allow for relaxed interactions; however, a sense of home can also be created by nurses and patients within any setting.

Thoughts of home may be ever present in the day to day dialogue between nurses and patients, and patients can be encouraged to express the value of home for them in story-telling and reminiscing. Nurses can encourage patients to align themselves with home, and together they can negotiate patients' usual home routines into the nursing care as much as it is possible.

Patients and nurses, who become so close to one another, develop a relationship which is best expressed as a 'family-like' tie. Nurses and patients can choose family-like relationships and risk the vulnerability of closeness, because they are not bound necessarily by the confines of a professional relationship, which might demand detachment.

Home is the most treasured place for people to be and nursing care can be geared towards helping people to return to their homes, if it is humanly possible. Nursing care can facilitate increasing independence and teaches coping skills, to the best of patients' abilities, so that they can return to their homes; however, nurses also assist patients to realise that they will never go home again.

Some practice possibilities of favouring

When patients and nurses are encouraged to recognise and approve commendable human qualities in each other, these expressions of approval can affirm these qualities as motivating forces with which to face the challenges of the day. Valuing and respecting each other then becomes something that assists nurse-patient relationships and fortifies their therapeutic potential.

Nurses work daily with people, doing their jobs to the best of their abilities, not expecting to receive statements of appreciation in return—but those offered are received with pleasure. The possibilities for practice here are related to the awareness that nursing is not only about giving, it can also be about receiving. Nurses can realise that it is OK to receive praise and gratitude from patients, and in so doing, to allow themselves to accept that they are worthy of those expressions.

Some practice possibilities of feelings

Nurses and patients can acknowledge the polarity of their human feelings, depending on what is happening for each individual. The possibilities for nursing practice here are related to the awareness that being happy or sad, being in comfort or pain, being relaxed or agitated, being calm or in fear, and being angry or content, are all natural consequences of living in a changeable world. This may require them to redefine their ideas about feelings in a way that they feel freer to share them sensitively with one another. The potential in this realisation is that the expression of feelings acknowledges the emotion and paves the way for clearer communication and appropriate actions.

Some practice possibilities of fun

Humour can soften the hard realities of people's circumstances and provide a means of levity, even temporarily, above the inevitability of certain ultimate tragedies. When humour is shared and sensitive to the other's situation, it can make people feel less lonely and connect them on lighter levels. Nurses and patients can enjoy some aspects of being together as people in health care contexts, even though the setting itself and the life circumstances of the patients may be relatively sombre and anxiety provoking. An awareness of the benefits of humour as a therapy in itself, can be a modality of care for nurses to explore and apply in their daily nursing practice.

Some practice possibilities of friendship

When nurses and patients take time to be together in nursing settings, they can begin to acknowledge the value of being there for one another for companionship and support. Patients value especially the time nurses spend with them talking and just being with them generally. Nurses can come to understand that sometimes company and talking are the most important things they can provide, as well as assisting patients with their activities of everyday living.

Some nurses and patients know each other so well that they feel and express affection and liking for each other. Affection comes from catching glimpses of each other as people, and it can extend past nursing settings to keeping connections with each other after the period of hospitalisation. Close ties with patients can create some personal emotional risks for nurses, especially as some patients will continue to be admitted until they finally succumb to their disease in death. Nurses who take the risks of close ties with patients can experience a fuller sense of knowing of the patient.

When nurses and patients take time and opportunities to get to know one another they can begin to understand the experiences of illness, as well as who and how they are as people, within their social networks, complete with their individual hopes and fears. Illness then becomes understood as more than just a physiological disturbance, and the person is seen as someone greater than a diagnostic label.

The common themes that permeate the qualities and activities and their possibilities for nursing practice are that the nurse-patient relationship is the focus of nursing's attention, that the development of this relationship occurs in contexts of care, and takes time and sensitivity to the other, and that the potential of the relationship is to improve patient care.

In as much as phenomenological research is directed towards a specific thing, in a certain place and time, and the meanings generated are always connected to the contextual features and understandings of its participants, this research cannot, and will not, attempt to generalise its meanings to other nursing settings. What can be raised, however, are possibilities for nursing practice. The effects of the phenomenon of ordinariness are those described through the methods and processes of this research, and if nurses recognise these enhancing potentials as relevant to their own practice, they may choose to put some of these ideas into action in their own professional experiences.

Insights for other health care professionals

What has been said of exploring nursing phenomenologically, in terms of its inability and unwillingness to generalise its findings, is true of any other application to health care professionals. The findings of this research cannot be transposed to other nurses and in their work places, nor can they be transposed to other professionals engaged in other forms of human health care services. However, what could happen for health professionals is that they could see some usefulness in the phenomenon of ordinariness, and use some these insights in their own practice.

Doctors, physiotherapists, occupational therapists, dietitians, social workers, dentists, and so on, could decide to humanise their approaches to their clients, by considering and embodying some or all of the aspects of facilitation, fair play, familiarity, family, favouring, feelings, fun, and friendship. To adopt these aspects in their professional practice would demonstrate that health professionals are willing to bring their ordinary human qualities and activities into their work worlds, as acknowledgment of the human status they share with their clients, thereby creating possibilities for enhancing these relationships.

Nurses and patients are the same in their humanity

Ordinariness in nursing refers to the sense of shared affinity that nurses and patients have for one another as humans. It is this sense of sameness as humans that gives them a common bond in the face of their individual existence as a nurse or a patient. The sense of sameness potentiates nursing as a caring and curing force in people's lives, and makes their stay in health care contexts manageable and familiar for them. This means that ordinariness in nursing is actually very important to nurses and patients and the development of their relationships, and that it is something that needs to be acknowledged as a positive contribution to patient care within the health care system.

The problem with such a pronouncement, of course, is that it appears initially that ordinariness in nursing is such a simple thing that it could not possibly have the degree of influence which this research is ascribing to it. This is the way of the world. When things appear familiar and apparently commonplace we may tend to take them for granted, and discount them as being relatively unimportant. The simple things can be among the most instructive agents in gaining wisdom and experience. I contend that ordinariness is one such case.

Reclaiming the potential of our human qualities of ordinariness

The qualities of being human that were described through the research process were common to the research participants, and it could be argued, that in a general sense, they are ways of seeing the potentiality of human existence. The actualities of allowingness, straightforwardness, self-likeness, homeliness, favourableness, intuneness, lightheartedness and connectedness, underlie aspects of living in the day to day world. The nature of these actualities may be so familiar that they are relatively invisible to the people in whom, and to whom, they are manifested.

If we consider the contingencies of everyday existence, successful interpersonal communication is no small feat. Negotiating the multitudinous features of living in a human world, replete with its symbols and circumstances, creates a veritable maze of unknowns and possibilities. When the challenges of daily life are considered, and the potentiality of humans to negotiate them are weighed up, the way becomes open to reconsider our human nature as qualities to be acknowledged, valued, and exercised.

Allowingness creates the potential for patients and nurses to help themselves, by providing some guidance and support until such a time, if at all, that people feel able to take over their own daily life business. Allowingness is considerate of the other person's needs to be independent and dignified; it helps quietly and carefully, always attentive to the cues within the other person that suggest a preparedness to resume increasingly autonomous thoughts and actions. Allowingness is possible in professional and personal life, whenever people are in a position of being of service to another person. This is no small thing; it is an act of thoughtfulness, directed towards the enhancement of one's own and the other person's existence.

Straightforwardness creates the potential for patients and nurses to speak to each other as frankly as possible, saying whatever it is that is in need of being said, at the same time tolerating each other's humanness. Straightforwardness is clear and concise in its delivery and generous in its intent; it speaks to the other to unblock impasses, and puts the perceived focus of contention plainly on view to trigger discussion. This human quality of straightforwardness and sensitive straight talking is manifested in professional and personal situations, when people need clear the air to create healthier communicative environments. This is no small thing; it is an act of courage, directed towards the enhancement of one's own and the other person's existence.

Self-likeness creates the potential for patients and nurses to understand the humanness of themselves in others, sharing an affinity as humans together, who are bonded by the commonality of their ordinary human existence. Through self-likeness people share a sense of togetherness, regardless of any differences they may happen to have. Self-likeness is possible in professional and personal life whenever people have the opportunities to relate to others as humans. This is no small thing; it is an act of sensitive relating, directed towards the enhancement of one's own and the other person's existence.

Homeliness creates the potential for patients and nurses to develop close interpersonal relationships, that encompass perspectives of people as family. Homeliness is sharing common understandings with people, and in so doing, accepting a share of their joys and pains, which are integral to closer human relationships. Homeliness is possible in professional and personal life whenever people have the opportunities to develop close interpersonal relationships. This is no small thing; it is an act of sensitive family-like bonding, directed towards the enhancement of one's own and the other person's existence.

Favourableness creates the potential for patients and nurses to give approval to other people and themselves and, in so doing, to magnify the attractive aspects of themselves. Favourableness is seeing beauty in people at the inside level; it recognises everyday human qualities that defy adequate description, and realises that it is only through sensing them within itself, that it is able to know that these qualities exist and how they are. Favourableness is possible in professional and personal life whenever people have opportunities to give approval to themselves and others. This is no small thing; it is an act of sensitive favouring, directed towards the enhancement of one's own and the other person's existence.

Intuneness creates the potential for patients and nurses to acknowledge and express the polarity of their feelings. Intuneness is clearing away the debris of rationality, to face up to, and embrace, the rawness of emotions, which when expressed, unblock the streams of human reactivity and cause our life energies to flow a little easier. Intuneness is possible in professional and personal life whenever people take opportunities to acknowledge and express their feelings. This is no small thing; it is an act of sensitive expressions of feeling, directed towards the enhancement of one's own and the other person's existence.

Lightheartedness creates the potential for patients and nurses to express themselves though humour, to lift themselves above their everyday circumstances. Lightheartedness is possible in professional and personal life whenever people take opportunities to engage in humour. This is no small thing; it is an act of sensitive humouring, directed towards the enhancement of one's own and the other person's existence.

Connectedness creates the potential for patients and nurses to know one another well enough to regard each other with affection. Connectedness is recognising friendly aspects in other people and coming in closer to get to know them. Connectedness takes time to get to know the other person, through keeping company and talking. Connectedness is possible in professional and personal life whenever people take opportunities to get to know one another affectionately. This is no small thing; it is an act of sensitive liking, directed towards the enhancement of one's own and the other person's existence.

The reciprocal nature of the actualities becomes evident in these descriptions of their potentiating energies. The apparently small and insignificant nature of everyday human qualities can take on a larger and more significant character, when they are seen as mutually enhancing forces in human life. The potentiating energies of the actualities are available to nurses and patients and, acknowledged, valued and exercised as something more than a familiar and commonplace phenomenon, ordinariness in nursing can become important and instructive in the daily work of nursing. Applied an a more general level to people, regardless of their connections with nursing, these human qualities can be acknowledged, valued, and exercised as mutually enhancing forces in interpersonal relationships. Regarded in this way, it becomes apparent that there may be value in reclaiming the potential of our human qualities of ordinariness in everyday personal and professional interpersonal encounters.

Nursing defined as what happens between nurses and patients in contexts of care

I began this book by noting that human interaction is about humans relating to one another in their respective worlds of other people and things. Nurses manage their daily nursing practice through human interactions, given their inclusion in people's lives when illness intervenes. Illness circumstances disrupt human relationships, in that they affect people and things. Illness either takes people away from their homes, or converts their homes into qualitatively different places. Home is a haven in which to feel safe and secure in its familiarity. Home is a place where daily routines go on, and body care is maintained, such as eating, sleeping, eliminating, hygiene, and so on. Home is where people perform private functions related to sexual needs and to other interpersonal intimacies. Home provides privacy and sanction to do such things as scratching private body parts, belching and breaking wind, and generally being basic, in a comfortable, non-public way.

It seems incongruent then, that at a time when people become ill and would probably benefit most from an increase in their private cathartic functions, they have to give up their respective private havens, to offer themselves up to relative control of health care institutions in the public domain. These places are not like home; they are populated with strangers providing services, most of whom are well-meaning, but none of whom is as familiar as family and friends at home.

The health care institutions seem to be full of professional people taking specific roles relating to body and mind care, a role for counselling, a role for resecting body parts, a role for regaining and maintaining muscle activity, a role for prescribing drugs and therapies, a role for almost everything, it seems. Of all the institutional health care populace, however, nurses appear to be the people in the greatest numbers and their roles seem less amenable to easy description somehow.

Nurses and patients are thrown together in random couplings, in places in which health care is managed as a service to the public. In their roles as registered health workers, nurses use their clinical knowledge and skills to give nursing care. The professional roles nurses occupy bear with them certain responsibilities and privileges, and even at the most minimal level nurses are expected to be wholly competent and polite.

While professional competence and politeness is standard behaviour for most people-oriented professions, it seems somewhat standard practice also that professionals forget, dismiss, or otherwise reject, their everyday genuineness as humans, when they engage in their professional contexts. Leaving their personal identities at home, health workers sally forth to their practice places each day to interact as masked professionals with the hapless inmates of the health care system.

Some nurses hide behind their professional masks in order to protect themselves from emotional knocks and bruises that result from clinical work, thus their professional facade acts as armour to protect them from the hurts of dealing with daily drama of human anguish. The roles of nurses and patients merge, and sometimes collide, in the immediacy and chaos of clinical settings. The challenge is for nurses to be themselves, in spite of the temptation to hide themselves away from the people who keep turning up in the roles of patients, complete with their stories of pain and challenge, day after day, year after year.

In their roles, nurses need to be alert to changes and react quickly to promote patient wellness. It is at this point that the acting metaphor becomes inadequate because, unlike actors, nurses in professional roles are responsible for their clinical decisions and behaviours. In acknowledging the importance of ordinary life roles, Goffman (1974) likened day to day life to performances of actors on a stage; but he claimed that actors have some protection against daily contingencies, unlike ordinary life in which people play out each moment as it comes.

Nursing is what happens between nurses and patients in contexts of care. The value of the nursing care is connected to the knowledge and skills with which nurses do their work, but it is also affected greatly by the way in which nursing care is given. It is the assertion of this book that the nurse-patient relationship is situated at the heart of what counts as nursing, and that this relationship is therapeutic when it dares to be human in the manner of its intent and actions in daily nursing encounters between nurses and patients.

As a practice discipline, nursing has struggled to explicate the nature of its work, and the effects that its practice has on people. I have argued elsewhere (Taylor, 1992a; 1992b) that many of the descriptions portraying nurses solely as professional helpers have robbed them of some of their inherent humanness and, thereby, have disconnected them from the very source of their human potential of caring and healing. Regardless of their professional role relationships and functions, nurse-patient relationships remain essentially human, embodying all the fundamentally ordinary qualities of people interacting in their worlds.

People are the reason for nursing's existence, and they hold the key to defining it in a way that encapsulates the nature of its existence. Nurses and patients are the same in their humanity, and it is this sameness that transcends any apparent differences they might have as individuals. The human qualities that were shown to be the actualities of the phenomenon of ordinariness have within them a generative force, which can be reclaimed by the awareness, valuing, and exercising of everyday human qualities. In view of these assumptions, my redefinition of nursing is simply this:

Nursing is what happens between nurses and patients in contexts of care, and it is facilitated by the humanity of both parties as they negotiate the illness experience together.

This does not mean, of course, that nursing is a simple practice and that any person can do it without prior knowledge or skills. Nurses are selected and educated carefully, to ensure that they are able to manage the demands of the work. I have argued elsewhere (Taylor 1991b, 1992b) that the absolute need for high standards of professional education and continuing practice are beyond doubt. What is being claimed here is that nurses are able to transcend the limitations of their professional roles and responsibilities to show themselves as human beings, who are proud of, and therapeutic through, the dynamic potential of their human simplicity.

The type of simplicity to which I refer is described well by Mary-Margaret Moore (1989), who provided a spiritual perspective of living the ordinary life, by suggesting that, as humans, our nature is love, and love is absolutely ordinary. She was careful to point out that she did not use the word ordinary to mean mediocrity, rather she used it in the sense of simple, as in uncomplicated. She suggested that:

> Ordinary is the answer. To be 'simple' in the moment will give you a sense of how you can just let go. In the letting go, your bound-up energy is released. The energy that is left can be used in a more creative way...By allowing yourself to experience the incredible wonder of the ordinary, you will create a space that allows other people to also be who they are. (p104)

Beyond ordinariness

In this concluding section I will extend the original findings of the research to suggest an ancient awareness, that is, that humans are spirit-filled beings, united in the extraordinary potential of their ordinary humanity. I used the metaphor of 'nurses as fairies in gumboots.' With absolutely no empirico-analytical proof what-soever, which is demanded by the objective world of hard science as the verifiability of truth, I claimed that humans are greater than they know because they are filled with spirit and that this makes them ultimately free. Rather like 'fairies in gumboots,' humans are interconnected, incarnate beings, with their feet weighted firmly to the ground.

Humans are earthed to daily routines and obligations that keep their attention to the apparent emotional polarities of life. In living their daily routines, they may have forgotten something of their spiritual heritage and their interconnectedness with all things but, thankfully, their forgetfulness is not entirely complete. The quality of their interpersonal relationships remind them now and then of the true beauty and power of their human existence.

I claimed that the awareness of spirit-filled existence is yet to strike the consciousness of many people on earth; but the awareness is growing, and it is facilitated to some extent through people-oriented vocations that seek to serve other human beings. Nurses are humans who, by service to others through nursing, have wonderful opportunities to be of use to themselves, to others, and to the planet. Nurses serve humanity through their clinical knowledge and skills, and it is through their human embodiment that they connect all other humans to themselves.

I used the experience of the research into ordinariness in nursing to claim that the work of clinical nursing contributes to therapeutic patient outcomes and attests to the value of nurses and patients being themselves as human beings, in the relatively strange context of the health care setting. Nurses' and patients' connectedness as humans transcends any professional differences they might have, and unifies them in the nurse-patient relationship so that the ordinariness of being human, defined as a sense of shared humanity (Taylor 1991a, 1992a, 1992b), becomes a powerful source of caring and healing. It is as though nurses and patients recognise one another as humans through a sensing that acknowledges, albeit implicitly, that they are spirit-filled beings, earthed in their gumboots of humanity, by their allowingness, straightforwardness, self-likeness, homeliness, favourableness, intuneness, lightheartedness, and connectedness (Taylor 1991a).

The effects of ordinariness can be therapeutic, so that nursing becomes known as a therapy in itself (McMahon & Pearson 1991). The therapeutic nature of nursing is related to the healing effects of nurses and patients interacting as humans together. Something more than nurses' knowledge and skills accounts for the healing effects, because the therapeutic effects are reciprocated between nurses and patients. Therapeutic nursing is related to the quality of the nurse-patient relationship and how this relationship mobilises healing responses in individuals. Therefore, valuing therapeutic nursing is the same as valuing the nurse-patient relationship as a potentiating force in health care.

The energising source of effective nursing

The nature of caring and curing in nursing has been explicated to some extent but, to date, no actual energising and enabling source of nursing has been suggested, other than the nature of human interaction itself. It is my bold assertion that nurses will know intuitively the source of the healing that comes through therapeutic nursing encounters. Healing is not necessarily slicing, dicing, testing, and ingesting; healing is caring, loving, accepting, and knowing with the inner heart in service to all. Healing is a human potential. To heal with the inner heart is simply a matter of 'returning home,' to remember and recognise the essence of one's humanness. 'Returning home' is listening to the inner voice of knowing, that knowing that hears the scholarly arguments of the empirico-analytical world, and says: "Yes, but..."

For some people like McFerrin (1988), the path homeward to the spirit within, is one they take without further ado; for others like Capra (1988) it is a matter of finding it through some form of rationality. In the Foreword of his little book entitled: *Don't Worry, Be Happy,* Bobby McFerrin (1988) writes these profoundly simple words:

I believe that life is fundamentally benevolent and people are basically good and know what's good for them. Things have a way of righting themselves without much meddling. No matter what those things are, big things, middle things, little things, I know we are bigger and greater than anything we meet along the way and we instinctively confront, bear down on and conquer anything that ails the collective soul. I know I'm part of everything. I'm part of nature and I know nature doesn't worry.

In his book *Uncommon Wisdom: Conversations With Remarkable People*, Fritjof Capra (1988) records a discussion he enjoyed with Ronald Laing about two seemingly different views of consciousness. They agreed that the Western scientific view of consciousness considers matter as primary, and consciousness as a property of complex material patterns that emerge by a process of biological evolution. The other main view is what may be called the mystical view, that consciousness is the primary reality, the essence of the universe, the ground of all Being, and everything else—all forms of matter and living beings are manifestations of pure consciousness. This view is based on non-ordinary modes of awareness, and as such it is regarded as indescribable.

When they considered an example of natural beauty, however, such as the place in which they stood as the sunset settled over the ocean, they agreed that its sights, sounds, and smells, were indescribable, and that not only mystical experiences, but also 'any experience of reality is indescribable' (Capra 1989 p142), because humans can take in the context of a single moment yet they are not able to describe fully that experience.

They proceeded to connect rationally the two seemingly different views of human consciousness.

The systems view of life agrees with the traditional scientific view, that consciousness is a property of complex material patterns, [precisely] a property of living things at a certain complexity. On the other hand, the biological structures of these systems are manifestations of under-lying processes...the process of self-organisation...identified as mental processes. In this sense, biological processes are manifestations of mind...[Extended]...to the universe as a whole, [it could be said] that all of its structures—from subatomic particles to galaxies and from bacteria to human beings—are manifestations of the universal dynamics of self-organisation, which means the cosmic mind. And this, more or less the mystical view. (p143).

Thus, Capra and Laing argued that the systems view of life can provide a meaningful framework for connecting the traditional approaches to questions of life, mind, and consciousness, and those put forward by the so-called mystical views. To get back to the original reason for this digression. McFerrin, Capra, and Laing have a sense of the connectedness of human consciousness, through their own ways of knowing. People may find a path homeward to the energising source of their humanness through a variety of means, such as the sacred writings (*The Bhagavadgita, The Koran, The Bible*), writings that are compilations of religious traditions (Hughes 1942, Rhys Davids 1956–1966, Waley 1958), so-called 'new age' publications (Houston 1990, Malone & Malone 1987, Millman 1992, Moore 1989) and, of course, the personal instruction that comes from the experience of one's own life. Each individual will know which is the best way for themselves.

The future of ordinariness for 'fairies in gumboots'

All people are 'fairies in gumboots,' in the sense that they are embodied spirit. What is the future for nurses, who are akin to 'fairies in gumboots?' I would like to suggest that, like all other humans, nurses are actually quite extraordinary in their ordinari-ness. Ordinariness of nursing is the shared affinity nurses and patients have for each other as humans. This humanness is not, as might be first thought, a small and inconsequential thing. I have attempted to show that the potentiality of human nature is an empowering force for nurses and patients, and for people generally.

Nurses are special in their uniqueness, a phenomenon often

forgotten, or taken-for-granted, in the familiarity of everyday embodied existence. Although some nurses may use actively in nursing their holistic perceptions and practices (Macrae 1985, Quinn 1985, Kreiger 1985, in Kunz 1985), it is my contention that a widespread acceptance and acknowledgment of nurses' humanness, the inherent spiritual essence of the humanity of nurses and patients, and the potentiality of that embodied spirituality, is not apparent in nursing writings and practice.

Even though Gardener (1982) might argue that these spirit-filled beings do in fact exist, I used the imagery of fairies in gumboots, as a metaphor to convey the meaning that, as 'fairies in gumboots,' humans are interconnected, incarnate beings, who have their feet weighted firmly to the ground. Humans are earthed to daily routines and obligations that keep their attention to the apparent emotional polarities of life. What was suggested was that humans are greater than they know. Humans are spirit-filled beings of love and light and, as such, they are a part of all there is. When humans gain a sense of their oneness, they need never feel small, insignificant, and lonely again. Humans are gaining a firmer and firmer sense of their spiritual heritage, thus the future looks bright for all people, and the healing of the planet. In nursing's particular interests, the future looks bright for nurses as 'fairies in gumboots' and for the work they do in their daily practice.

This natural extension of ordinariness in nursing is, in part, nothing new; it is simply the reiteration of an old age awareness, put into a New Age context. Simply stated it is this: there are interconnections between all people, and in the embodied nature of the nurse-patient relationship the 'magic' that is brought about by those sparks of spirit (Capra 1988, Moore 1989) unites nurses and patients as one with each other and their environment. In this sense, humans are all one with all there is. There is no separation.

Closing comments

This book has given a description of the considerations, stories and meanings, that comprise the phenomenon of ordinariness in nursing. It was offered as a user-friendly version of my PhD thesis, to give some understandings of how I came to define ordinariness and, in so doing, to offer a redefinition of nursing. The redefinition is simplicity itself, because people are the reason for nursing, and they hold the key to defining it in a way that encapsulates the nature of its existence. Stated simply it is that:

Nursing is what happens between nurses and patients in contexts of care, and it is facilitated by the humanity of both parties, as they negotiate the illness experience together.

Nurses and patients are the same in their humanity and it is this sameness, that transcends any apparent differences they might have as individuals. The generative force of humanness can be reclaimed simply by the awareness, valuing, and exercising of it. Aspects of ordinariness such as facilitation, fair play, familiarity, family, favouring, feelings, fun and friendship can have advantageous effects. Nurses and patients can sense an affinity as humans and they negotiate the illness experience together through their human qualities of allowingness, straightforwardness, self-likeness, homeliness, favourableness, intuneness, lightheartedness, and connectedness. Ordinariness is sophisticated in its simplicity. The shared human qualities of nurses and patients have within them the generative source of humanness, which is the ability to care for, and cure, one another.

Bibliography

Aamodt A M 1983 Problems in doing nursing research: developing a criteria for evaluating qualitative research. Western Journal of Nursing Research 5398–402

Abdellah F G, Beland I L, Martin A, Matheney R V 1960 Patient-centered approaches to nursing. Macmillan, New York

Adeloytte M K 1985 Nursing's societal discontent and societal change. In: Wieczorek R R (ed) Power politics and policy in nursing. Springer, New York

Aho W R, Minott K 1977 Creole and doctor medicine: folk beliefs practices and orientations to modern medicine in a rural and an industrial suburban setting in Trinidad and Tobago the West Indies. Social Science and Medicine 11:349–355

Allen D 1985 Nursing research and social control: alternative models of nursing that emphasise understanding and emancipation. Image 17 (2):58–64

Allen D, Benner P, Diekelmann N L 1986 Three paradigms for nursing research: methodological implications. In: Chinn P L (ed) Nursing research methodology: issues and implementation. Aspen, Rockville

Anderson J M 1981 An interpretive approach to clinical nursing research. Nursing Papers 13(4):6–12

Anderson J M 1987 Cultural context of caring. Canadian Critical Care Nursing 4 (4):7–13

Angeles P A 1981 Dictionary of philosophy. Barnes & Noble, New York

Asuni T 1979 Dilemma of traditional healing with special reference to Nigeria. Social Science and Medicine 13(1):33–39

Author unknown 1985 Folk medicine still used. Occupational Health Nursing 33(4):108–9

Author unknown 1986 Alternative medicine: bridging the gap. Nursing (UK) 3(12):461–465

Author unknown 1988 An a-z of natural therapies. The Lamp 44(10):20–5

Banonis B C 1989 The lived experience of recovering from addiction: a phenomenological study. Nursing Science Quarterly 2:37–43

Barbee E L 1986 Biomedical resistance to ethnomedicine in Botswana. Social Science and Medicine 22(1):75–80

Beckstrand J 1978a The notion of a practice theory and the relationship of scientific and ethical knowledge to practice. Research in Nursing and Health 1(3):131–136

Beckstrand J 1978b The need for a practice theory as indicated by the knowledge used in the conduct of practice. In: Nicoll L H (ed) Perspectives on nursing theory. Scott Foresman, Illinois

Beckstrand J 1980 A critique of several conceptions of practice theory in nursing. Research in Nursing and Health 3(2):69–80

Benner P 1983 Uncovering the knowledge embedded in clinical practice. Image: Journal of Nursing Scholarship 15(3):36–41

Benner P 1984 From novice to expert: uncovering the knowledge embedded in clinical practice. Addison-Wesley, California

Benner P 1985 Quality of life: a phenomenological perspective on explanation prediction and understanding in nursing science. Advances in Nursing Science 8(1):1–14

Benner P, Wrubel J 1989 The primacy of caring: stress and coping in health and illness. Addison-Wesley, California

Benoliel J 1984 Advancing nursing science: qualitative approaches. Western Journal of Nursing Research Summer 6(3):1–8

Bergum V 1989 Being a phenomenological researcher. In: Morse J M (ed) Qualitative nursing research: a contemporary dialogue. Aspen, Maryland

Bhagavadgita, The. Translated fron the Sanskrit with an introduction by Juan Mascaro 1962 Penguin Books, Baltimore

Boxall J F 1988 Sayings and superstitions. Midwives Chronicle and Nursing Notes Dec: 400

Brown L 1986 The experience of care: patient perspectives. Topics in Clinical Nursing 8 (2):56–62

Brown J 1989 Emancipation through praxis: the reflexive relationship between theory and practice. National Nursing Theory Conference School of Nursing Studies, Sturt, South Australian College of Advanced Education

Buber M 1958 I and thou, 2nd edn. (Smith R G trans.) Charles Schribner's Sons, New York

Buber M 1965 Distance and relation. (Smith R G trans.) In: Friedman M (ed) The knowledge of man. Harper & Row, New York

Bulbrook M J 1984 Health and healing in the future. The Canadian Nurse Dec:26–29

Bullock A, Stallybrass O, Trombley S (eds) 1988 The Fontana dictionary of modern thought, 2nd edn. Fontana Press, London

Campbell A V 1984 Moderated love: a theology of professional care. Photobooks, Bristol

Campbell A V 1985 Paid to care: the limits of professionalism in pastoral care. Anchor Press, Great Britain

Capers C F 1985 Nursing and the Afro-American client. TCN 7(3):11–17

Capra F 1988 Uncommon wisdom: conversations with remarkable people. Fontana Paperbacks, London

Carper B A 1978 Fundamental patterns of knowing in nursing. Advances in Nursing Science 1:13–23

Carr W, Kemmis S 1984 Becoming critical: knowing through action research. Deakin University Press, Victoria

Carstairs G M 1977 Knowers of charms. New Society 40(763):336–337

Cate P 1986 Bach flower remedies. Health Visitor 59:276–277

Chinn P L 1985 Debunking myths in nursing theory and research. Image xvii(2):45–49

Chinn P L, Jacobs M K 1987 Theory and nursing: a systematic approach, 2nd edn. Mosby, St Louis

Chinn P L 1988 Nursing patterns of knowing and feminist thought. Nursing and Health Care, February

Chinn P L, Jacobs M K 1983 The emergence of nursing theory. Mosby, St Louis

Chinn P L, Kramer M K 1991 Theory and nursing: a systematic approach, 3rd edn. Mosby Year Book, St Louis

Christman L 1983 The future of nursing is predicted by the state of science and technology. In: Chaska N (ed) The nursing profession: a time to speak. McGraw-Hill, New York

Christman N J, Johnson J E 1981 The importance of research in nursing. In: Williamson Y M (ed) Research methodology and its application to nursing. Wiley, New York

Colaizzi P 1978 Psychological research as the phenomenologist views it. In: Valle R S, King M (eds) Existential phenomenological alternatives for psychology. Oxford University Press, New York

Conway M E 1985 Toward greater specificity in defining nursing's metaparadigm. Advances in Nursing Science July:73–81

Cooper P 1984 Drugs and herbal remedies. Midwife Health Visitor and Community Nurse 1:16

Crow R 1982 Frontiers of nursing in the twenty-first century. Journal of Advanced Nursing 7:111–116

Culbertson J A 1981 Three epistemologies and the study of educational administration. Review, The University Council for Educational Administration 22(1):1–6

Curtin L L 1987 About nurses: perceptions and misperceptions. Nursing Management 18(1):11–12

Darbyshire P 1985 Bedpans or broomsticks? Nursing Times Nov:44–5

Davis A 1973 The phenomenological approach in nursing research. In: Garrison E (ed) Doctoral preparation for nurses. University of California, San Francisco

Davis A 1978 The phenomenological approach in nursing research. In: Chaska N (ed) The nursing profession: views through the mist. McGraw-Hill, New York

Derrida J 1983 Speech and phenomena and other essays of Husserl's theory of signs. Northwestern University Press, Evanston

Descartes R 1970 The philosophical works of Descartes. (Haldane E S, Ross G R T trans.) Cambridge University Press, Cambridge

Diers D 1979 Research in nursing practice. Lippincott, Philadelphia

Dilthey W 1985 Poetry and experience. Selected works, Vol V. Princeton University Press, New Jersey

Dobbs B Z 1985 Oncology nursing: alternative health approaches. Nursing Mirror 160(9):41–2

Donaldson S, Crowley D M 1978 The discipline of nursing. Nursing Outlook February:113–120

Douglas J D 1974 Understanding everyday life. Routledge and Kegan Paul, London

Dreyfus H I 1979 What computers can't do: the limits of artificial intelligence. Harper & Row, New York

Dreyfus S E, Dreyfus H L 1980 A five-stage model of mental activities involved in directed skill acquisition. Unpublished report supported by the Air Force Office of Scientific Research, University of California, Berkeley

Dreyfus H L 1991 Being-in-the-world: a commentary on Heidegger's being and time. Division 1, The MIT Press, Cambridge, Massachusetts

Drew N 1986 Exclusion and confirmation: a phenomenology of patients' experiences with caregivers. IMAGE: Journal of Nursing Scholarship 18 (2):39–43

Dring S 1985 Old wives tales: eye of newt... Community Outlook Dec:12–3

Dunlop M 1986 Is a science of caring possible? Journal of Advanced Nursing 11:661–670

Dunlop M 1988 Science and caring: are they compatible? shaping nursing theory and practice: the Australian context, La Trobe University, Lincoln School of Health Sciences: Department of Nursing, Melbourne

Eisenberg L 1977 Disease and illness: distinctions between professional and popular ideas of sickness. Culture Medicine and Psychiatry 1(1):9–23

Ellerton N, Downe-Wamboldt B 1987 Concerns of hospice patients and the role of hospice volunteers. Journal of Palliative Care 3(1):16–22

Erickson H C, Tomlin M, Swain M A 1983 Modeling and remodeling: a theory and paradigm for nursing. Prentice-Hall, Englewood Cliffs

Farber M 1947 Concerning freedom from presuppositions. Philosophy and Phenomenological Research 7:367–368

Fawcett J 1984 Analysis and evaluation of conceptual models of nursing. F A Davis, Philadelphia

Fawcett J 1989 Analysis and evaluation of conceptual models of nursing, 2nd edn. F A Davis, Philadelphia

Field P, Morse J 1985 Nursing research: the application of qualitative approaches. Croom Helm, London

Fitzpatrick J J, Whall A L 1989 Conceptual models of nursing: analysis and application. Appleton and Lange, Connecticut

Flanagin A 1989 (ed) Sanitation spirits and medicine: health care in the African bush. JAMA 261(8):1–1202

Flew A 1986 David Hume: philosopher of moral science. Basil Blackwell, Oxford

Fook J 1988 Teaching casework: incorporating radical and feminist perspectives in the curriculum. In: Advances in social welfare education. University of New South Wales, Sydney

Forbes H A W 1985 Alternative health care: selected individual therapies. New Zealand Nursing Journal 78(3):27–9

Forrest D 1989 The experience of caring. Journal of Advanced Nursing 14:815–823

Frederick H, Northam E 1938 A textbook of nursing practice. Macmillan, New York

Fromm E 1956 The art of love. Harper & Row, New York

Gadamer H-G 1975 Truth and method. Barden G, Cumming J (ed and trans.) Seabury, New York

Gadamer H-G 1976 The universality of the hermeneutical problem. Philosophical hermeneutics. (Linge D E trans) University of California Press, Berkeley

Gadow S 1980 Existential advocacy. In: Spiker S F, Gadow S (eds) Nursing: ideas and images opening dialogue with the humanities. Springer, New York

Gardner L E 1982 Pictures of fairies: the Cottingley photographs. First Quest Edition, Theosophical Publishing House, Wheaton, Illinois

Gartrell E G 1987 Women healers and domestic remedies in the 18th century America: the recipe book of Elizabeth Coates Paschall. New York State Journal of Medicine, 87(1):23–9

Gino C 1985 Rusty. A true story. Pan Books, London

Giorgi A, Fischer C L, Murray E L 1975 Duquesne studies in phenomenological psychology. Pittsburgh, Duquesne University Press, 2

Glittenberg J 1974 Adapting health care to a cultural setting. American Journal of Nursing, Dec:2218–2221

Goffman E 1961 Encounters: two studies in the sociology of interaction. Bobbs-Merrill, Indianapolis

Goffman E 1974 The presentation of self in everyday life. Pelican Books, London

Goldstein D (undated) A traditional navajo woman...a modern midwife...healing in harmony. Frontier Nursing Service, Quarterly Bulletin: 7–13

Gortner S 1983a The history and philosophy of nursing science and research. Advances in Nursing Science Jan: 1–8

Gortner S 1983b Knowledge in a practice discipline: philosophy and pragmatics. Keynote Address American Academy of Nursing Meeting, Minneapolis, Minnesota

Gray G, Pratt R (eds) 1991 Toward the discipline of nursing. Churchill
    Livingstone, Melbourne
Green E C 1985 Traditional healers, mothers and childhood disease in
    Swaziland: the interface of anthropology and health education. Social
    Science and Medicine 2(3):277–285
Gregory D, Stewart P 1987 Nurses and traditional healers: now is the time to
    speak. The Canadian Nurse Sept: 25-27
Gulino C K 1982 Entering the mysterious dimensions of others: an existential
    approach to nursing care. Nursing Outlook 30(6):352–357
Habermas J 1972 Knowledge and human interests. Heinemann, London
Hall L E 1964 Nursing: what is it? The Canadian Nurse
    60(2):150–154
Hall A L, Bourne P G 1973 Indigenous therapists in a southern black urban
    community. Arch Gen Psychiatry 28 Jan:137–142
Harris J 1980 The contribution of non-professionals in psychiatric care. Nursing
    Times April 3:602–603
Heidegger M 1962 Being and time. (Macquarrie J, Robinson E trans.)
    Harper & Row, New York
Hekman S J 1986 Hermeneutics and the sociology of knowledge. Polity Press,
    Cambridge
Helman E 1986 An autumn life: how a surgeon faced his fatal illness.
    Faber & Faber, London
Henderson V1955 Textbook of principles and practice of nursing. Macmillan,
    New York
HendersonV 1966 The nature of nursing. Macmillan, New York
Hillman A 1986a Zone therapy. Nursing (Oxford) 3rd Series 3(6):225– 7
Hillman A 1986b Zone alternative medicine: an introduction, Part 1 Nursing
    (Oxford) 3rd Series 3(1):26–8
Houston J 1990 The search for the beloved: journeys in sacred pychology.
    J P Tharcher, Los Angeles
Hughes E R 1942 The great learning and the meaning-in-action: newly
    translated from the Chinese, with an introductory essay on the history of
    Chinese philosophy. J M Dent, London
Husserl E 1960 Cartesian meditations: an introduction to phenomenology.
    (Cairns D trans.) Matinus Nijhoff, The Hague
Husserl E 1964 The idea of phenomenology. (Alston W P, Nakhnikian G trans.)
    Martinus Nijhoff, The Hague
Husserl E 1965 Phenomenology and the crisis of philosophy. (Lauer Q trans.)
    Harper & Row, New York
Husserl E 1970 The crisis of the European sciences and transcendental
    phenomenology. Northwestern University Press, Evanston
Husserl E 1980 Phenomenonology and the foundations of the sciences.
    (Klein T E, Pohl W E trans.) Martinus Nijhoff, The Hague
Hyde A 1977 The phenomenon of caring, Part VI. American Nurses'
    Foundation 12(1):2
Jegede R O, Williams A O, Sijuwola A O 1985 Recent developments in the care,
    treatment, and rehabilitation of chronically mentally ill in Nigeria. Hospital
    and Community Psychiatry 36(6):658–61
Johnson D E 1968 Theory in nursing: borrowed and unique. Nursing Research
    17(3):206–209
Johnson D E 1980 The behavioural system for nursing. In: Riehl J P,
    Roy C (eds) Conceptual models for nursing practice, 2nd edn.
    Appleton-Century-Crofts, New York
Jourard S M 1971 The transparent self. D Van Nostrand, New York
Kant E 1929 A critique of pure reason. (Kemp Smith N trans.) Macmillan,
    London

Karlsson E L , Moloanetea K E A 1986 Traditional healer in primary health care: yes or no? Nursing RSA Verpledging 1(2):26–9

Kelly K 1985 Nurse practitioner challenges to the orthodox structure of health care delivery: regulation and restraints on trade. American Journal of Law and Medicine 11(2):195–225

Kemp V A 1983 Themes in theory development. In: Chaska N L (ed) 1983 The nursing profession: a time to speak. Mc Graw-Hill , New York

Kestenbaum V 1982 (ed) The humanity of the ill: phenomenological perspective. University of Tennessee Press, Knoxville

King I M 1971 Toward a theory for nursing: general concepts of human behaviour. John Wiley, New York

King I M 1981 A theory for nursing: systems concepts process. John Wiley, New York

Kinlein M L 1977 Independent nursing practice with clients. Lippincott, Philadelphia

Kitson A L 1984 Steps towards the identification and development of nursing therapeutic functions in the care of hospitalised elderly. Unpublished PhD thesis, University of Ulster, Coleraine

Kleiman S 1986 Humanistic nursing: the phenomenological theory of Paterson and Zderad. In: Winstead-Fry (ed) 1986 Case studies in nursing theory. National League for Nursing, New York

Kleinman A 1977 Explaining the efficacy of indigenous therapies: the need for interdisciplinary research. Culture Medicine and Psychiatry 1:133–134

Kleinman A 1978a Concepts and a model for comparison of medical systems as cultural sytstems. Social Science and Medicine 12:85–93

Kleinman A 1978b Problems and prospects in comparative cross-cultural medical and psychiatric studies. In: Kleinman A, Kunstadter P, Alexander E R, Gale J L (eds) Culture and healing in Asian societies. Schenkman, Cambridge

Knaack P 1984 Phenomenological research. Western Journal of Nursing Research 6:107–114

Knowledge in nursing 1988 Study guide. Deakin University, Geelong

Kockelmans J J 1967 (ed) Phenomenology: the philosophy of Edmund Husserl and its interpretation. Doubleday, New York

Koran, The. Translated from the Arabic with notes by N J Dawood, (4th edn) 1974 Penguin, Hammondsworth

Krell D F 1977 Martin Heidegger: basic writings. Harper and Row, New York

Kretlow F 1990 A phenomenological view of illness. Australian Journal of Advanced Nursing 7(2):8–10

Kunz D 1985 Spiritual aspects of the healing arts. Theosophical Publishing House, Wheaton, Illinois

Kvale S 1984 The qualitative research interview: a phenomenological and hermeneutical mode of understanding. Journal of Phenomenological Psychology 14(2):171–96

Laing R D 1967 The politics of experience. Ballantine, New York

Lamb R M 1987 Healing: examining the perspectives. Journal of Holistic Nursing 5(1):23–26

Langveld M J 1978 The stillness of the secret place. Phenomenology and Pedagogy 1(1):181–189

Lawler J 1991 Behind the screens: nursing, somology and the problem of the body. Churchill Livingstone, Melbourne

Leddy S, Pepper J M 1989 Conceptual bases of professional nursing, 2nd edn. Lippincott, Philadelphia

Lee P A 1986 Traditional medicine: dilemmas in nursing practice. Nursing Administration Quarterly Spring: 14–20

Leininger M 1979 Transcultural nursing. Masson Publishing, New York
Leininger M 1985 Qualitative research methods in nursing. Grune & Stratton, New York
Levine M 1971 Holistic nursing. Nursing Clinics of North America, 6(2) June:253–264
Levine M E 1973 Introduction to clinical nursing, 2nd edn. F A Davis, Philadelphia
Lopez P, Getzel G S 1987 Strategies for volunteers caring for persons with AIDS. Social Casework 68(1):47–53
Lumby J 1991 Nursing: reflecting on an evolving practice. Deakin University Press, Geelong
Lye Chng C, Kirby Ramsey M 1984 Volunteers and the care of the terminal patient. Omega 15(3):237–244
Mackenzie M 1987 The alternative patient. Nursing Times 83(25):36–9
Malone T P, Malone P T 1987 The art of intimacy. Prentice-Hall, New York
Marriner A 1986 Nursing theorists and their work. Mosby, St Louis
Marriner-Tomey A 1989 (ed) Nursing theorists and their work. 2nd edn. Mosby, St Louis
Mayeroff M 1971 On caring. Harper and Row, New York
McFerrin B 1988 Don't worry, be happy. Dealacorte Press, New York
McMahon R, Pearson A (eds) 1991 Nursing as therapy. Chapman & Hall, London
McPherson P 1987 The quality of being expressed as doing. The Australian Journal of Advanced Nursing, 5(1):38–42
Meleis A I 1985 Theoretical nursing: development and progress Lippincott, Philadelphia
Meleis A I 1986 Theory development and domain concepts. In: Moccia P (ed) 1986 New approaches to theory development. National League for Nursing, New York
Merleau-Ponty M 1962 Phenomenology of perception. Routledge & Kegan Paul, London
Merleau-Ponty M 1964 The primacy of perception and other essays on phenomenological psychology. Northwestern University Press, Evanston
Merleau-Ponty M 1967 What is phenomenology? In: Kockelmans J J (ed) Phenomenology: the philosophy of Edmund Husserl and its interpretation. Doubleday, New York
Mitchell G J 1990 The lived experience of taking life day-by-day in later life: research guided by Parse's emergent method. Nursing Science Quarterly: 29–36
Millman D 1992 No ordinary moments: a peaceful warrior's guide to daily life. H J Kramer, Tiburon, California
Moccia P (ed) 1986 Theory development and nursing practice: a synopsis of a study of the theory-practice dialectic. New Approaches to Theory Development, National League for Nursing, New York
Moore M-M 1986 Bartholomew: I come as brother. High Mesa Press, Taos
Moore M-M 1989 Bartholomew: reflections of an elder brother. High Mesa Press, Taos
Morris M 1977 An excursion into creative sociology. Columbia University Press, New York
Morse J M (ed) 1989 Qualitative nursing research: a contemporary dialogue. Aspen, Rockville
Motlana N 1988 Tryanny of superstition. Nursing RSA Verlpeging 3(1):17–9
Muetzel P A Therapeutic nursing. In: Pearson A 1988 (ed) Primary Nursing. Croom Helm, London
Munhall P, Oiler C J (eds) 1986 Nursing research: a qualitative perspective. Appleton-Century-Crofts, Norwalk

Netting F E , Thibault J M 1986 Using volunteers with the elderly in health care settings. The Journal of Applied Gerontology 5(2):139–152

Neuman B M 1982 The Neuman systems model: an application to nursing education and practice. Appleton-Century-Crofts, Norwalk

Neuman B 1989 The Neuman systems model. Appleton & Lange, Norwalk, Connecticut

New English Bible, The. 1971 Cambridge University Press, New York

Newman M A 1979 Theory development in nursing. F A Davis, Philadelphia

Nicoll L H 1986 Perspectives on nursing theories. Little, Brown, Boston

Nightingale F 1893 1955 In: Selected writings of Florence Nightingale (Compiled by Seymer L). Macmillan, New York

Nightingale F 1859 1980 Notes on nursing: what it is and what it is not. Churchill Livingstone, Edinburgh

Noddings N 1981 Caring. Journal of Curriculum Theorizing 3(2):139–148

Norris C M 1982 Concept clarification: evolving methods in nursing. Concept clarification in nursing. Aspen, Maryland

Obediyi A I, Togonu-Bickersteth F 1987 Concepts and management of deafness in the Yoruba medical system: a case of traditional healers in Ile-Ife Nigeria. Social Science and Medicine 28(4):645–649

O'Grady A 1989 Past life therapy. Paper presented at the proceedings of the 10th National Homebirth Conference, Sydney

Oiler C 1982 The phenomenological approach in nursing research. Nursing Research 31(3):171–181

Oiler C 1986 Phenomenology: the method. In: Munhall P, Oiler C J (eds) 1986 Nursing research: a qualitative perspective. Appleton-Century-Crofts, Norwalk

Olsson K 1989 Caribou bones and labrador tea. The Canadian Nurse Feb:18–21

Omery A 1983 Phenomenology: a method for nursing research. Advances in Nursing Science 5(2):49–63

Orem D 1959 Guides for developing curricula for the education of practical nurses. Government Printing Office, Washington, D C

Orem D E 1985 Nursing: concepts of practice, 3rd edn. McGraw-Hill, New York

Orem D E 1987 Orem's general theory of nursing. In: Parse R R 1987 Nursing science: major paradigms theories and critiques. W B Saunders, Philadelphia

Orlando I J 1961 The dynamic nurse-patient relationship. Putnam's, New York

Orr J A 1979 Nursing and the process of scientific enquiry. Journal of Advanced Nursing 4(6):603–610

Osis M (undated) Herbal remedies: food for thought. Gerontion: 8–11

Palmer D 1988 Looking at philosophy: the unbearable heaviness of philosophy made lighter. Mayfield, California

Parker J 1986 Shifts in Australian nursing education In: Proceedings of the International Nursing Conference: Destiny of Nursing. Nashville, Tennessee

Parker J M 1988 Theoretical perspectives in nursing: from microphysics to hermeneutics. Third Nursing Research Forum, Lincoln School of Health Sciences, La Trobe University, Melbourne

Parse R R 1981 Man-living-health: a theory of nursing. John Wiley, New York

Parse R R 1985 Nursing research: qualitative methods. Brady, Bowie

Parse R R 1987 Nursing science: major paradigms theories and critiques. W B Saunders, Philadelphia

Parse R R 1990 Parse's research methodology with an illustration of the lived experience of hope. Nursing Science Quarterly: 9–17

Parse R R, Coyne A B, Smith M J 1985 Nursing research: qualitative methods. Brady, Bowie

Patchner M A, Finn M B 1987–88 Volunteers: the life line of hospice. Omega: An International Journal of Dying and Death 18(2):135–144

Paterson J 1971 From a philosophy of clinical nursing to a method of nursology. Nursing Research March-April 20(2):143–146

Paterson J G 1978 The tortuous way toward nursing theory. In: Theory development: what why how? National League for Nursing, New York

Paterson J, Zderad L 1976 Humanistic nursing. Wiley, New York

Patton M G 1980 Qualitative evaluation methods. Sage Publications, Beverley Hills, California

Pearson A 1983a What the public thinks. Nursing Times Feb 23:18–19

Pearson A 1983b Primary nursing. Nursing Times Oct 5:37–38

Pearson A 1984a A centre for nursing. Nursing Times July 18:52–54

Pearson A 1984b The essence of advanced nursing is being there. Nursing Mirror Sept 4:16

Pearson A 1984c The Burford experience. Nursing Mirror Dec 12: 32-35

Pearson A 1985a Introducing new norms in a nursing unit and an analysis of the process of change. Unpublished PhD thesis, Department of Social Science and Administration, University of London

Pearson A 1985b The Burford experiment. Paper presented at the European Conference on Advanced Clinical Practice. Barbican Centre, London

Pearson A 1985c The Burford experience. Paper presented at the Society of Nurses in Advanced Practice Conference, Wrexham

Pearson A 1985d Nursing beds in the British NHS. Paper presented at the University of Manchester, Department of Nursing, 25th Anniversary Conference, Manchester

Pearson A 1986a The unique role of the nurse. Senior Nurse 6(4):45–49

Pearson A 1986b Introducing new norms in a nursing unit—an action research study, Paper presented to the Oxford Regional Research Interest Group

Pearson A 1987a Who's in charge here? In: Clinical judgement and decision making: the future with nursing diagnosis (conference proceedings). John Wiley, Canada

Pearson A 1987b Nurse controlled units: an innovation in medical-surgical nursing. Paper presented to the Advances in Medical-Surgical Nursing Conference, New York

Pearson A 1988a Just an ordinary nurse. Lakeside graduation address. (unpublished)

Pearson A 1988b Nursing: from whence to where. Professorial Lecture, Deakin University, Geelong

Pearson A 1988c (ed) Primary nursing. Croom Helm, London

Pearson A 1988d Primary nursing—nursing in the Oxford and Burford nursing development units Croom Helm, London

Pearson A 1988e Nursing beds—an alternative health care provision. Oxfordshire Health Authority, Oxford

Pearson A 1988f Therapeutic nursing—the effects of admission to a nursing unit. Oxfordshire Health Authority, Oxford

Pearson A 1988g Developing the practice of nursing. Paper presented to Fellows and Members of the New South Wales College of Nursing, February

Pearson A 1988h Therapeutic nursing: the effect of admission to a nursing unit on patient outcome. Paper presented to Future Directions Conference, SA Health Commission, Adelaide, August

Pearson A 1989 Translating rhetoric into practice: theory in action. National Nursing Theory Conference, School of Nursing Studies, Sturt, South Australian College of Advanced Education

Pearson A 1990a Therapeutic nursing: transforming models and theories in action. In: Akinsanya, J A (ed) Recent advances in nursing: theories and models for nursing. Churchill Livingstone, London

Pearson A 1990b Therapeutic nursing. Paper presented at the Adelaide Children's Hospital, March

Pearson A 1992a Nursing at Burford—a story of change. Scutari Press, London

Pearson A 1992b Knowing nursing: emerging paradigms in nursing. In: Vaughan B, Robinson K (eds) Knowledge for nursing. Heinemann, London

Pearson A, Durand I, Punton S 1988a The feasibility and effectiveness of nursing beds. Nursing Times 84:48–50

Pearson A, Durand I, Punton S 1988b Effects of admission to a nursing unit. Australian Journal of Advanced Nursing, 6 (Sept-Nov):38–42

Pearson A, Durand I, Punton S 1989 Determining quality in a unit where nursing is the primary intervention. Journal of Advanced Nursing 14:269–273

Pearson A, Durand I, Punton S 1992 Nursing beds: an evaluation of therapeutic nursing. Scutari Press, London

Pearson A , McMahon R 1991 Nursing as therapy. Chapman Hall, London

Pearson A, Vaughan B 1986 Nursing models for practice. Heinemann Nursing, London

Peplau H E 1952 Interpersonal relations in nursing. Putnam, New York

Potterton D 1983 Culpeper and his cure-alls. Health and Social Science Journal 93:154–6

Psathas G 1973 Phenomenological sociology: issues and applications. John Wiley, New York

Ranin M 1978 Non-traditional health care practices. Alaska Nurse 27(5):6–7

Rhys Davids T W 1956–1966 Dialogue of the Buddha. In: Sacred books of the Buddhists. (translated from the Pali) Luzac, London

Rickman H P (ed) 1976 Wilhelm Dilthey: selected writings. Cambridge University Press, Cambridge

Riehl J P, Roy C 1980 Conceptual models for nursing practice. Appleton-Century-Crofts, New York

Rieman D J 1986 The essential structure of a caring interaction: doing phenomenology. In: Munhall P, Oiler C J (eds) 1986 Nursing research: a qualitative perspective. Appleton-Century-Crofts, Norwalk

Robertson M H B 1987a Home remedies: a cultural study. Home Health Care Nurse 5(1):35–40

Robertson M 1987b Folk health beliefs of health professionals. Western Journal of Nursing Research 9(2):257–63

Rogers M 1961 Educational revolution in nursing. Macmillan, New York

Rogers M E 1970 The theoretical basis of nursing. F A Davis Company, Philadelphia

Roper N, Logan W W, Tierney A J 1980 The elements of nursing. Churchill Livingstone, Edinburgh

Rosenblum E H 1980 Conversation with a Navajo nurse. American Journal of Nursing August: 1459–1461

Rosser A 1982 Every witch way herbal remedies. Nursing Mirror 155(17):20–2

Roy C 1976 Introduction to nursing: an adaptation model. Prentice-Hall, Englewood Cliffs

Sanda A O 1978 Scientific or magical ways of knowing: implications for the study of African traditional healers. Second Order 1-2:70–84

Scheiermacher F 1977 Hermeneutics: the handwritten manuscripts. (Kimmerle H ed), Scholars Press, Atlanta

Schwartz H, Jacobs J 1979 Qualitative sociology: a method to the madness. Free Press, New York

Scott Verinis J 1970 Therapeutic effectiveness of untrained volunteers with chronic patients. Journal of Consulting and Clinical Psychology 34(2):152–155

Searle C 1980 The power of the folk healer. International Cancer Nursing Conference 5, 125(23):30–4

Silva M, Rothbart D 1984 An analysis of the changing trends in philosophies of science on nursing theory development and testing. Advances in Nursing Science January 6 (2)

Silverman H 1984 Phenomenology: from hermeneutics to deconstruction. Research in Phenomenology XIV:19–34

Singer C 1959 A short history of scientific ideas to 1890. Oxford University Press, London

Smith M C 1984 Research methodology: epistemologic considerations. Image: Journal of Nursing Scholarship xvii (2):42–46

Smyth J 1986 The reflective practitioner in nurse education. Proceedings of the Second National Nursing Education Seminar: Visions into Practice. South Australian College of Advanced Education, Adelaide

Spiegelberg H 1970 On some human uses of phenomenology. In: Smith F J (ed) Phenomenology in perspective. Martinus Nijhoff, The Hague

Spiegelberg H 1975 Doing phenomenology. Martinus Nijhoff, The Hague

Spiegelberg H 1976 The phenomenological movement, Vols I and II. Martinus Nijhoff, The Hague

Spradley J P 1980 Participant observation. Holt Rinehart Winston, New York

Stapleton T J 1983 Husserl and Heidegger: the question of a phenomenological beginning. State University of New York Press, Albany

Steiner G 1978 Heidegger. Fontana Press, London

Stevenson E W, Viney L L 1973 The effectiveness of nonprofessional therapists with chronic psychotic patients: an experimental study. Journal of Nervous and Mental Disease 156(1):38–45

Stewart D, Mickunas A 1974 Exploring phenomenology: a guide to the field and its literature. American Library Association, Chicago

Street A 1990 Nursing practice; high hard ground messy swamps and the pathways in between. Deakin University Press, Geelong

Street A 1991 From image to action: reflection in nursing practice. Deakin University Press, Geelong

Sukale M 1976 Comparative studies in phenomenology. Martinus Nijhoff, The Hague

Suppe F, Jacox A 1985 Philosophy of science and the development of nursing theory. In: Werley H H, Fitzpatrick J J (eds) Annual review of nursing research, Springer, New York

Swaffield L 1988 Communication: tuned in. Nursing Times 84(23):28–31

Swanson J M, Chenitz W C 1982 Why qualitative research in nursing? Nursing Outlook April: 241–245

Swanwick T 1986 Alternative medicine: bridging the gap. Nursing 3(12):461–465

Taylor B J 1988 What are the patients' perceptions of the usefulness of information given to them by nurses and what are the nurses' perceptions of their roles and constraints as teachers in giving effective patient education in a postnatal ward? A research paper submitted in partial fulfilment of the requirements for the degree of Master of Education, Deakin University, Geelong

Taylor B J 1990 Journalling: towards critically self-reflective practice. In: Study guide, searches for meaning in nursing 2: cultural meanings and practices in nursing. Deakin University Press, Geelong

Taylor B J 1991a The phenomenon of ordinariness in nursing. Unpublished PhD thesis, Deakin University, Geelong

Taylor B J 1991b The dialectic of the nurse as person: ordinary nurses perceived as extraordinarily effective. Conference proceedings: Science Reflectivity and Nursing Care: Exploring the Dialectic, Melbourne

Taylor B J 1992a Relieving pain through ordinariness in nursing: a phenomenologic account of a comforting nurse-patient encounter. Advances in Nursing Science 15(1):33–43

Taylor B J 1992b From helper to human: a reconceptualisation of the nurse as person. Journal of Advanced Nursing 17:1042–1049

Tilden V P, Tilden S 1985 The participant philosophy in nursing science. Image: Journal of Nursing Scholarship 17(3):88–90

Tinkle M, Beaton J 1983 Towards a new view of science. Advances in Nursing Science Jan: 27–36

Thomas J 1988 Kill or cure. Nursing Times 8(7):39–40

Thompson J L 1987 Critical scholarship. Advances in Nursing Science 10(1)27–38

Torres G 1986 Theoretical foundations of nursing. Appleton-Century-Crofts, Norwalk, Connecticut

Torrey E F 1969 The case for the indigenous therapist. Arch Gen Psychiat 20 March

Travelbee J 1963 What do we mean by rapport? American Journal of Nursing February 63:725–728

Travelbee J 1966 Interpersonal aspects of nursing. F A Davis, Philadelphia

Travelbee J 1971 Interpersonal aspects of nursing. F A Davis, Philadelphia

Treece E W, Treece J W 1977 Elements of research in nursing. Mosby, St Louis

Tripp-Reimer T 1983 Retention of a folk healing practice (matiasma) among four generations of urban Greek immigrants. Nursing Research 32(2):97–101

Turton P 1986 Joining forces. Nursing Times Nov 19:31–32

Tutton E 1991 An exploration of touch and its use in nursing. In: McMahon R, Pearson A (eds) Nursing as therapy. Chapman & Hall, London

Unit NPR 305 Searches for meaning in nursing 1: phenomenon encountered in nursing. Bibiliography document 1993, Deakin University, Geelong

Van Kaam A L 1959 The nurse in the patient's world. American Journal of Nursing 59(12):1708–1710

Van Kaam A 1959 Phenomenological analysis: exemplified by a study of the experience of being really understood. Individual Psychology 15:66–72

Van Kaam A 1969 Existential foundations of psychology. Doubleday, New York

Van Manen M 1978–79 An experiment in educational theorising: he Utrecht school. Interchange 10(1):48–66

Van Manen M 1984 Doing phenomenological research and writing: an introduction. University of Alberta, Edmonton

Visintainer M A 1986 The nature of knowledge and theory in nursing. Image: Journal of Nursing Scholarship 18(2):32–38

Warner R 1977 Witchcraft and soul loss: implications for community psychiatry. Hospital and Community Psychiatry 28(9):686–90

Waley A 1958 The way and its power: a study of the Tao te ching and its place in Chinese thought. Grove Press, New York

Watson J 1979 Nursing: the philosophy and science of caring. Little Brown, Boston

Watson J 1981 Nursing's scientific quest. Nursing Outlook 29(7):413–416

Watson J 1988 Nursing: human science and human care: a theory of nursing. National League for Nursing, New York

Weaver M T 1985 Acupressure: an overview of theory and application. Nurse Practitioner 10(8):38–42

Westwood C 1986 Aromatherapy. Health Visitor 59:251

Wiedenbach E 1964 Clinical nursing: a helping art. Springer, New York

Winstead-Fry P 1980 The scientific method and its impact on holistic health. Advances in Nursing Science Jan: 1–7

Wolf J H 1985 Professionalising volunteer work in a black neighbourhood. Social Service Review 59(3):423–434

Wooding C 1983 Afro-Surinamese case study on paralysis and voodoo death. Curare 6(1):13–24

Workshop Report Document 1989 School of Nursing, Deakin University, January

Zaner R 1970 The way of phenomenology: criticism as a philosophical discipline. Pegasus, New York

Zaner R M 1970 The way of phenomenology. Bobbs-Merrill, Indianapolis

Zaner R 1971 The problem of embodiment: some contributions to a phenomenology of the body. Martinus Nijhoff, The Hague

Index